A QUESTION OF CHOICE

A Question of Choice

Bioethical Reflections on a Spiritual Response to the Technological Imperative

PAM McGRATH

Routledge
Taylor & Francis Group
LONDON AND NEW YORK

First published 1997 by Ashgate Publishing

Reissued 2018 by Routledge
2 Park Square, Milton Park, Abingdon, Oxon, OX14 4RN
711 Third Avenue, New York, NY I 0017, USA

Routledge is an imprint of the Taylor & Francis Group, an informa business

A Library of Congress record exists under LC control number: 97074821

ISBN 13: 978-1-138-60892-4 (hbk)
ISBN 13: 978-0-429-45994-8 (ebk)

Contents

Acknowledgements

I would like to express my gratitude to my close friends Meg and Geoff Waugh, not only for the energy they placed into formatting and proof reading this text, but also for the warmth and support they have shown to me over the years.

My appreciation also goes to my valued friend Dr Christopher Newell for his enthusiastic support for this project.

Finally, I would like to extend a special thank you to my lovely daughters Amy, Emma, Zoe and Bo. The privilege of being your mother has nourished and energised me throughout the difficult time of researching and completing this book. Without your love and support this work would not have been possible.

Preface

This research wishes to make a contribution to our understanding about 'the way' our society responds to issues of death and dying. Situated within the discipline of bioethics, this research used postmodern notions of discourse and power to explore one, local, organisational response to working with the dying - that of the Karuna Hospice Service, (KHS).

In modern, western, technological societies, biomedicine is the dominant discourse which underpins our care of the terminally ill. Bioethics has recently emerged as a discipline concerned with resolving the many ethical dilemmas arising from such a physiological, technologised approach to death. Rather than add to such studies, this research looked in the direction of alternative 'ways' of responding to the dying within our community. KHS was chosen for this research as it presented the possibility of a holistic and spiritual alternative to the positivist, reductionist, mechanistic hegemony of scientific medicine. This research, then, was concerned with establishing and describing this difference, and exploring how such an organisation of 'difference' could maintain resistance to mainstream biomedicine.

The outcome of this inquiry is a detailed description and interpretation of the uniqueness of this service, its process of coming into existence and the ongoing negotiation of its legitimacy to practice in the health arena. Central to the discussion of all the understandings that emerged from this research is the acknowledgment of a spiritual dynamic that underpins the discursive practices of this organisation. Such a spiritual dynamic is seen to impact on all aspects of this service, from defining its difference to facilitating and maintaining its existence. Consequently, this notion of spirituality became the central concern of this research.

In our society, because of the dominance of secular modernist ideas of rationalism and positivistic science, notions of spirituality have been at best, marginalised, and at worst, excluded from our discourse on death and dying. Research into spirituality has been limited by modernist epistemological assumptions concerning proof and measurement. This work seeks to make a contribution to the reversal of such a direction by offering an example of research which is inclusive of the notion of spirituality. It is argued that an anti-foundational postmodern *episteme* provides ways of thinking differently about, and hence researching, such metaphysical issues. By shifting from concerns about truth to notions of discourse, this postmodern research was able to explore the ideas of spirituality which emerged in the discursive practices of Karuna Hospice Service.

It will be argued that, in this spiritual discourse, there are constructive, proactive ingredients which could inform our work with the dying. The 'will-to-care', the provision of choice, the acceptance of difference and a taoist response to power are all important aspects of KHS's discourse which can enrich our understanding of alternative 'ways' of responding to the many problems arising from the biomedical model and the 'technological imperative' that drives it. Consequently, it will be the conclusion of this research that the spiritual discourse of KHS has important implications for both the disciplines of bioethics and palliative care.

1 Introduction

> When Daedalus, who can be thought of as the master technician of most ancient Greece, put the wings he had made on his son Icarus, so that he might fly out of and escape from the Cretan labyrinth which he himself had invented, he said to him; 'Fly the middle way. Don't fly too high, or the sun will melt the wax on your wings, and you will fall. Don't fly too low, or the tides of the sea will catch you'. Daedalus himself flew the middle way, but he watched his son become ecstatic and fly too high. The wax melted, and the boy fell into the sea. For some reason, people talk more about Icarus than about Daedalus, as though the wings themselves had been responsible for the young astronaut's fall. But that is no case against industry and science. Poor Icarus fell into the water - but Daedalus, who flew the middle way, succeeded in getting to the other shore (Campbell, 1988:131-2).

These insights, which Campbell draws from an ancient Greek myth, introduce and underpin both the subject matter and the direction of this research. It evokes a questioning of the interrelationship between humans and the creative extension of their life world known as technology. Such a questioning will focus in particular on the recent and extensive intrusion of technology, in the form of medicalized care, into the way our society responds to those who are dying.

This exploration of the interface between technology[1] and the human experience of dying will be situated within the recently emerged discipline of bioethics. This discipline presently focuses predominantly on the normative concern of how to resolve difficult moral, practical and legal issues arising from our extensive use of technology in health matters.[2] In this case, the exploration of these ethical issues will be contextualized to end-of-life situations. The assumption is that this myth provides the starting point with its questions about direction and its reflection on concerns about 'the way'. The suggestion is not that, when faced with issues of dying in the context of technologised twentieth century medicine, there is a 'middle way', or even that we have begun to articulate the parameters of 'the other shore'.

In short, the concern will be with exploring 'the ways' our society responds to issues of death and dying.

Exploring new directions in bioethics

A great deal of work has been published about the way our society handles death and dying. This work has primarily been situated in the dominant (first order) discourse of the biomedical model (Freund and McGuire, 1991:226-228; Turner, 1987), and the 'technological imperative' that drives it (Fuchs, 1968). As the intent of the present discussion is to explore new directions this dominant discourse and its implications for death and dying (Martocchio 1982:25; Munley, 1983:11) will only be taken as a starting point to operate as an intertextual reference for later discussions.

Although for this work biomedicine will be viewed as but one, albeit dominant, discourse, it is important to note that there is a direct and significant relationship between the historical development of bioethics and this first order discourse. Indeed, as Jonsen notes (1990:57) the discipline of bioethics arose in the 1960s as a response to the increasingly complex ethical and legal issues, resulting from modern western technologised medicine's invasion into all areas of human life eg., conception, birth, life and death.

In 1961, a major advance in the technology of kidney dialysis at the Seattle Artificial Kidney Centre, in the form of an arteriovenous shunt, paved the way for a clinically useful artificial kidney machine - a life saving device for many individuals. The resulting problem was that resources for this extensively useful technology were limited. Decisions had to be made about who could and who could not be accepted for treatment. Hence, the discipline of bioethics was born (Jonsen, 1990:18), and the issue of resource allocation has been a central issue ever since.

The term 'bioethics' is taken from the Greek word, *bios,* meaning 'life', and thus can be understood as ordinary ethics applied to the 'bio-realm' (Johnstone, 1994:31). It has been defined by the International Association of Bioethics as 'the study of ethical, social, legal and other related issues arising in health care and the biological sciences' (Singer, 1993:298). As articulated by Johnson, bioethics 'deals not only with how we treat patients in a medical sense, but also how we relate to, or deal with, our fellow human beings, especially in matters of illness, injury, dying and death' (1990:338). The present research into end-of-life issues fits well into these parameters.

Bioethical discourse is predominantly preoccupied with resolving problems which arise from the use/abuse of technology in biomedical interventions in health issues. Understandably, criticism has been levelled at the discipline of bioethics because it appears to be trapped in the minutiae of clinical decisions which legitimise present medicocentrism (Fox, 1994).[3] Such a restricted approach is seen to be oblivious to the social and cultural context in which these decisions occur (Weisz, 1991:3).[4]

The focus has been micro-ethical, with reflection restricted to a philosophical concern about how to respond to ethical dilemmas after they arise, in the context of clinical practice.[5] This approach ignores or minimises a dialogue on the wider picture, which would incorporate a sociological understanding of how such dilemmas originate.

Changing directions

My previous postgraduate research for a Master of Arts, titled, 'Chemotherapy: Treatment, Experimentation or Illusion', is located easily within the above description, as it examined issues arising from the reductionist, biomedical, 'state-of-the-art' discourse in relation to cytotoxic drug use in cancer treatment. This research explored the many ethical problems arising from the extensive, and at times, inappropriate use of this modality in oncology. Such problems included the ethical dilemmas created by the toxicity of the drugs used, the lack of underlying scientific theory, the problems with efficacy, and the lack of consideration for the effect of such drug use on the patient and family (McGrath, 1992; 1996; McGrath & Markman, 1996).

Central to understanding such issues was a consideration of the impact of the western, scientific, linear nature of research in this area, with its clinical focus on the 'battle with cancer', rather than a holistic consideration of the patient's needs (McGrath, 1993).

This research into chemotherapy, understandably, touched on insurmountable problems associated with the power of medical dominance, the entrenched scientific, bio-medical paradigm, the influence of the drug industries, and unrealistic media 'hype' about 'breakthroughs' in drug research (McGrath, 1995; McGrath and Kearsley, 1995; McGrath and Turner, 1995).

Much as I enthusiastically embraced publishing and speaking on the findings of the research, I hungered for a positive perspective: a constructive response to the dilemmas of the 'hi-tech medical fix'. Although I was aware that highly technologised, clinical medicine, based on scientific theoretical foundations, was the dominant model (Zola, 1990; Turner, 1987; Fairclough, 1992:3), the assumption was not made that it was the *only* model.[6]

It was during this time of disseminating my findings on the ethics of chemotherapy that I was introduced to the work of Karuna Hospice Service (henceforth referred to as KHS). With a growing sense of delight and satisfaction, I began to understand the excellent work of this service.

Instead of duplicating the many studies on the first order (dominant) discourse of biomedicine, I decided instead to explore the possible contribution of an alternative discourse. Consequently, through the privilege of being involved with this organisation, I undertook a different direction of exploring alternative 'ways' of responding to the needs of the dying.

The strategy I developed was to step outside the grand narrative of reductionistic, technologised, western medicine, to explore 'other ways' of handling end-of-life situations. My intention was not to contribute to the mass of very valuable research relevant to bioethics which has already been conducted on the milieu of modern, technologised medicine.[7] Rather, this work is predicated on the assumption that in the face of the enormous body of research on the biomedical model, and in view of the fact that little work exists on alternative approaches to end-of-life issues, such as Karuna Hospice Service (Siebold, 1992:158), it is important to look in new directions.

A caveat to seeking a new direction, however, is that such a searching does not mean a rejection, *carte blanche,* of the medical model. The concern is with exploring the possibilities inherent in a dialogue that accommodates both the positives in allopathic medicine and the contribution of an intervention (which will be shown to be) based predominantly on a spiritual understanding.

A central motivation for this research, then, is a desire to move away from a bioethical approach based on analysing the minutiae of clinical decision making in a technologised process. The important assumption underpinning such a move is an acknowledgement that the biomedical approach is but one social construction of reality: albeit, a dominant one[8] with the epistemological and political power capable of limiting other ways of understanding. Rather than accepting such a view of reality, with its knowledge claims disguised as 'truth', the concern will be to challenge such an understanding with an exploration of other 'ways' of knowing.

The challenge is to move outside the truth-production of the biomedical model and examine other possibilities for understanding and responding to end-of-life ethical issues. Such an approach incorporates and values an understanding of 'housekeeping' issues (i.e. a concern with developing satisfying and constructive environments as a way of responding to ethical issues), as opposed to 'crisis' practices (Holmes and Purdy, 1992:3). This is based on the assumption that it is better to examine the epistemological and sociological processes impacting on a situation, rather than to simply react to a crisis when the situation becomes unmanageable.

The central questions such research wishes to explore are - Does a different way of thinking and talking about death and dying actually translate into different actions and decisions? If so, are there proactive ingredients in the discourses running through KHS, which could promote beneficence, and act in a preventative way to deter the complicated, and difficult to resolve, ethical dilemmas that now dominate the bioethical discourse?

An individual facing a terminal illness within our society will, through a process both within and outside their control, become involved in a therapeutic milieu philosophically determined by prevailing discourses. For the majority that will mean the institutional care provided by biomedicine;[9] for a few, the holistic care of a community based hospice service. The 'difference' between these alternative milieus is the central focus of this research.[10]

Why Karuna?

Karuna Hospice Service (KHS), a community based palliative care service which works with the dying provides an example, it is suggested, of one such alternative to the bio-medical model.

As the main reason for choosing KHS is because it is seen as a constructive, effective and positive alternative practice for working with the dying, it is important to indicate the sources of information, which provided my provisional observation that KHS was in fact, such an alternative. I was aware of -

1 Enthusiastic stories by families who had received support from KHS in the process of coping with a family member who had died.

2 Positive reports from past and present members of the KHS organisation about the satisfaction with their work within the service. Such satisfaction was expressed not only with Karuna's philosophy, as different from the bio-medical model, but also with the opportunity that this organisation provided to achieve positive, work-related goals.

3 Newspaper articles on KHS which provided anecdotal information with regards to a satisfying experience with dying.

4 Feed-back from health professionals, and allied health professionals, outside the organisation, who have had dealings with this service, and have affirmed with enthusiasm this service's constructive and creative contribution to terminal care.

Such sources of information were not to be taken as an indication, *tout court,* that Karuna was unquestionably a successful, alternative enterprise. Rather, they provided the promise that Karuna may potentially offer discourse examples different from the institutional biomedical model when focused on the issues of death and dying.

What is Karuna?

KHS is a recently formed (May, 1991), community based hospice organisation, which provides comprehensive home care services for people with a life-threatening illness and their families. The administration for this service is situated in a modest, fibro building that is part of the previous Rosemount Psychiatric hospital, Windsor, Brisbane. This small, eight- roomed building is immaculately kept and simply furnished. Decorated with a few posters and the occasional Buddhist artefact, this building provides an ambience which is both welcoming and non-threatening. At present, the building is of sufficient size to accommodate this small service.

As it is a Buddhist based hospice with a Buddhist monk as director, this service differs from the usual hospice by not having a physician as either director or full-time member of staff. KHS carries out most of its work in the community (although admissions to hospital and in-patient hospices can be arranged). Nurses, trained in palliative care and transported in cars provided by the Queensland Cancer Fund, provide the support necessary for patients who choose to spend their remaining life at home. Specially trained volunteers are available for companionship and respite care. Bereavement counselling and support is provided by trained workers, for families in the year following the patient's death.

The stated rationale for KHS's service is underpinned by the notion of choice, as outlined in the leaflet on their service which reads,

> By taking hospice care into the home, Karuna provides people with a choice. Our aim is to ensure that people with terminal illnesses, and their families, enjoy the highest quality of remaining life.

The research focus

The starting assumption for generating this research was that KHS's approach is outside the hegemony of mainstream medicine. As a Buddhist, community based organisation that works with the dying without a medical director (or even a physician employed part-time), it is viewed as having a difference that may challenge the selective interests of the prevailing medical status quo. The initial expectation was that 'such discourses are likely to be marginal to existing practice and dismissed by the hegemonic system of meanings and practices as irrelevant or bad' (Weedon, 1987:35). It is the relationship between these two different discourses, one dominant and one marginal, that is the crucial focus. According to postmodern analysis (as will be detailed in later chapters), the effects of power can be isolated and articulated where differing discourses meet (Perakyla, 1989:131).

This research originally sought to establish whether KHS was, indeed, a service with a difference. Hence, the initial focus was on the question of the uniqueness of Karuna Hospice Service. This exploration was developed with the secondary questions in mind of - How this uniqueness (if documented), is sustained in relation to the biomedical model? and, What constructive contribution such an alternative model could offer to our approach to death and dying in our society? An implicit assumption in such questioning was a belief that KHS offered a discourse of resistance to the dominant, technologised, scientific discourse on dying within our society. Researchers in hospice care, such as Siebold (1992:138), record that community based hospices (such as KHS), in comparison to those hospices that were an extension of medical institutions, had far greater difficulty in negotiating their existence and surviving. Questions, then, of how KHS maintained its resistance to the 'high-tech' medical model became the second major focus of this work.

It is important to point out at this stage that no comparison will be made between KHS and other hospices (either locally or world wide). To make such a comparison would necessitate extending the research (focus, methodological framework and data collection) to include the discourses of other hospices. Such a process is clearly beyond the scope of the present research.

Within this focus, *uniqueness* and *resistance* were the original key words of interest that underpinned the research and raised the following questions -

1 What is the uniqueness of Karuna hospice service?

2 What are the discourses on dying running through the Karuna hospice service? If these discourses indicate a difference to other discourses on dying within our society, in particular the bio-medical discourse, how does it resist the hegemonic power of such discourses?

It must be stressed at this stage that these questions formed the initial or preliminary research assumptions for this work. As will be discussed later, these assumptions were subsequently reformulated during the research process.

Postmodern ideas, in particular notions of discourse and deconstruction, constitute the basic philosophical lens for this research. It will be the task of the following chapter to begin to explore these postmodern notions. Before doing so, however, a chapter summary will be provided to make the development of ideas throughout this book as clear as possible.

Book summary

This introductory chapter situated the research in the discipline of bioethics. The reasons for choosing to explore alternative ways of responding to bioethical concerns arising from the care of the dying were discussed through reflections on my previous postgraduate work in this area. The organisation that will be the focus of this study, Karuna Hospice Service, was introduced and briefly described. The research questions and the rationale for choosing this service were provided.

Chapter two explores in detail the many postmodern notions which underpin this research. The discussion moves from a critique of modernist research methodology to an exploration of the constructive possibilities in the postmodern approach. The notions arising from the postmodern literature on discourse and power are presented as ideas central to understanding the direction of this research. This focus on discourse and power, combined with the use of ideas formulated by writers on deconstruction are outlined as the central approach to research. The potentiality for criticisms with regards to such an approach will be anticipated, acknowledged and responded to with constructive suggestions.

Chapter three applies the theoretical notions introduced in the previous chapter to an exploration of the research method adopted for this study. This detailed discussion incorporates descriptive information on the participants, the production of data and the research process. Such a discussion includes an explanation of why language/texts were used and how they were developed for data collection (which entails an analysis of the process of engaging in non-directive interviewing as the medium used for the development of these language/texts). This chapter concludes with a discussion on the steps followed in developing an analysis of this data.

Chapter four begins the task of sharing with the reader a description of the material collected. The focus is on the first research question, concerned with establishing KHS's difference from other organisations working with the dying. The next four chapters are concerned with situating this stated difference within the significant discourses running through this organisation. This chapter ends by introducing the first of such discourses, that of Hospice/Palliative care, and shows how the 'talk' of KHS can be situated within the conceptual understanding of the international hospice movement.

Chapter five introduces the second significant discourse for consideration: KHS's Buddhist discourse. This Buddhist 'talk', which is based on central notions of compassion and wisdom and focuses on the significance of death and dying, is shown to be similar to, and compatible with, the previously discussed hospice discourse.

Chapter six moves the discussion from the specific Buddhist metaphysic to a more generic discourse on spirituality which arises from the language/texts. The primacy of this spiritual discourse to KHS is emphasised. The notion that such a discourse will be interpreted as the cardinal dynamic underpinning and energising this organisation's 'difference' and 'resistance' to biomedicine, is introduced. This 'gentle' spiritual discourse of tolerance and caring is shown to be compatible with, and supportive of, the other significant discourses running through this organisation.

As each of these major discourses is to some degree informed by the more generic, modern, western discourse on death and dying, the focus of chapter seven turns to an examination of this discourse. The 'talk' of KHS, situated at the interface of the Hospice, Buddhist and Spiritual discourses, is shown to be involved in a constructive response to the more troubling notions of the highly technologised, reductionist, scientific, western approach to death and dying.

Chapter eight recognizes how KHS's difference was not only defined in terms of what it is, but sometimes in terms of what it is not. Such statements of contrast referred to the biomedical model. Consequently, this chapter explores in detail many of the assumptions that underpin this model and the technological imperative that drives it.

Having established KHS's difference to biomedicine, chapter nine begins the exploration of how this service managed to establish its existence with such a powerful and dominant discourse. This is the beginning of the interpretative (as different to the previously descriptive) analysis of this research. The assumption is made explicit that such existence was not assured and that, as a community based hospice without a medical director, such a project would be seen to be most unlikely to succeed. The threats to KHS's establishment are explored, setting the stage for the discussion of how these obstacles are overcome.

Chapter ten situates the language/texts which relate to KHS's successful negotiation with the system in the context of hospice development world wide. The story which unfolds is one of a strong charismatic leader, with a vision imparted by his Buddhist teacher, who brings together a network of dedicated and highly respected professionals and hard working volunteers, who through 'sheer blood sweat and tears' eventually manage to negotiate public funding and an excellent reputation. Such a story resonates with the hospice literature. In spite of its stated difference, an analysis of this process highlights the conservative notions underpinning its success. The notion of an 'exemplary counter-institution' is used to interpret KHS's successful adaption.

The story of KHS's resistance does not end with the granting of public funding. Such funding brings with it demands for professionalisation and bureaucratisation, which challenge the spiritual vision of this service. This challenge to spiritual goals is shared by hospices world wide. Chapter eleven explores how this service continues to negotiate its difference in the face of demands from mainstream medicine. Using Weberian theoretical notions of the move from charismatic movement to routinisation (professionalism and bureaucratisation), KHS's accommodation to such demands is interpreted as inevitable. Although KHS's spiritual discourse is seen to inevitably defer to such power (interpreted in this discussion as rationalisation to the system), its Taoist (going with the flow) rather than oppositional relationship to power is shown to provide a considerable influence in protecting this organisation from the full power of the system. In short, KHS's spiritual discourse is shown to be a creative response to the inevitable encroachment of the power of mainstream health care.

Chapter twelve continues the exploration of KHS's creative spiritual response. Although it is acknowledged that this organisation's psycho-spiritual discourse is easily dominated by hegemonic notions of professionalism and bureaucracy, it is argued that, when translated into a particular form of subjectivity at the organisational level, it could be seen as a point of considerable resistance. The discourses of this organisation are seen to create a 'spiritual space' whereby the individual, in spite of the demands from more powerful discourses, can choose to act with difference. KHS's spiritual discourse is seen to shape a subjectivity which attracts and supports individuals who are comfortable with a gentle, caring, tolerant, and dedicated way of seeing the world. Such individuals are supported organisationally to engage in holistic care of the dying. This is contrasted with the subjectivity of the biomedical model. Of importance is the understanding that different discourses are shown to translate into different subjectivities and hence different 'ways' of caring for the dying.

Chapter thirteen draws together the above outlined insights into KHS's different way of caring for the dying and reflects on the implication of such findings for the discipline of bioethics. With a focus on the notion of choice, this chapter suggests that the spiritual discourse of KHS could inform our present understanding of end-of-life bioethical dilemmas by the pragmatic demonstration of a different 'way' of responding to the care of the dying.

In consideration of the postmodern tenet that in the text only the reader speaks, the concluding chapter (fourteen) takes the opportunity to explore the possibility of other readings of this research material.

Notes

1 Cassell defines technology as 'the modalities and instrumentalities that greatly extend the *power* of human action, sensation, or thought in ways that are *independent* of the particular user' (Author's emphasis, 1993:32). Such a definition has been chosen because it suggests the tension between the promise of power and the Frankensteinian sense of a force independent of its creator. This is an ongoing theme throughout the literature on the human experience of technology.

2 The noted ethicist, Callahan, summarises and articulates this central concern of most bioethicists that biomedicine's technology is strongly implicated in creating such end-of-life dilemmas when he writes that 'enhanced biological knowledge and technological skill have served to make our dying all the more problematic: harder to predict, more difficult to manage, the source of more moral dilemmas and nasty choices, and spiritually more productive of anguish, ambivalence and uncertainty' (1993:33).

3 The nub of concern over such a restricted perspective (ideas which will be developed fully in later discussions) is, as Weisz's (1991) points out, the lack of a broader sociological or historical appreciation of the genesis of such problems. According to Weisz, 'there is something about the way these issues are usually handled which seems somehow inappropriate if not wrong-headed to one trained in a discipline like sociology or history. In their analysis of complex situations, ethicists often appear grandly oblivious to the social and cultural context in which these occur, and indeed to empirical referents of any sort' (1991:3).

4 This exclusive concern with clinical issues can be seen by the following brief summary of topics considered of interest to bioethics. The subject matter and questions asked are an extension of the biomedical definition and control of health, which include such issues as: the stress of diagnostic technology (Best, 1987; Daly, 1989; Green et al., 1993; Kearsley and Hirst, 1991; King, 1987; Lazarus and Leeder, 1989; Lerman et al., 1991; Lowe, 1989; MacDonald, 1989; Taylor, 1986; Walker et al., 1989), the use of drugs (Dutton, 1988; Kessler, 1991; Klein, 1992; McGrath, 1992; McGrath, 1993; McGrath, 1995; McGrath and Kearsley, 1995; Ratcliff, 1989), the permanent vegetative state (King, 1987), artificial hearts (Dutton, 1988), genetic engineering (Dutton, 1988), Invitro Fertilisation (Donchin, 1989; Dunstan and Shinebourne, 1989;Lorber, 1989; Ratcliff, 1989) defining death (Thomson, 1982) experimentation (Coney, 1988; Johnstone, 1994; Jones, 1989), transplantation (Johnstone, 1994; Shaw et al., 1991; Teo, 1991) technologised neonatal care (Dunstan and Shinebourne, 1989) Intensive Care Units (Fairman, 1992; Dunstan and Shinebourne, 1989; Ratcliff, 1989), the excessive costs of technology (King, 1987; Leeder, 1989; Lowe, 1989; Melski, 1992; Rutten and Bonsel, 1992; Williams, 1992) and treatment refusals or withdrawing treatment (Emanuel et. al., 1991; Edwards and Tolle, 1993; Evans and Brody, 1985; Devereux, Jones and Dickenson, 1993; Fisher and Raper, 1990; Johnstone,

1994; Kliever, 1989; McInerney, 1992; Sabatino, 1993; Scofield, 1991a; Tomlinson and Brody, 1988). Such issues arise directly from the present highly technologised medicocentric practices in health care.

5 This exclusive concern with philosophical reflection (called Principlism) will be dealt with in detail in later chapters. Suffice here to provide Green's findings (1990:180) that the primary method in bioethics is a reasoned evaluation of normative arguments that typifies the field of moral philosophy. Bioethics, defined by Green, 'involves the self-critical application of modes of moral reasoning, in the form of ethical theory or fundamental moral principles, to the new range of questions raised by the biomedical sciences.'

6 As will be discussed in detail in later chapters, this model is structured around the power of the medical profession: a phenomenon known as 'medical dominance' (Willis, 1994:17; 1989). Karuna Hospice Service, is situated well outside this model as it does not employ a physician and was founded by a Buddhist physiotherapist.

7 From a transdisciplinary perspective there is a wealth of writings and research on the biomedical model that informs bioethics (Aaron and Schwartz, 1984; Aaron and Schwartz, 1985; Almond, 1988; Andrews, 1986; Armstrong, 1987; Bates and Birch, 1981; Bates and Lapsley, 1985; Bedell et al., 1983; Berliner, 1984; Black, 1988; Bok, 1976; Borges, 1986; Brody, 1989; Cairns, 1978; Carr-Gregg and Hobbs, 1988; Cassell, 1991a; Cassell, 1991b; Kliever, 1989; Crawshaw, 1983; Dellaport, 1987; Dochin, 1989; Dutton, 1988; Faulder, 1985; Fisher, 1991; Fox, 1993; Fuchs, 1968; Goodin, 1988; Hewa and Hetherington, 1990; Illich, 1976; Jecker, 1991a; Jennett, 1992; Jensen and Mooney, 1990; Johnstone, 1994; Jones, 1988; Jonsen, 1990; Kennedy, 1981; Klein, 1992; Kogan, 1991; Leeder, 1989; Maseide, 1991; Mishler, 1981; Miyaja, 1993; Navarro, 1986; Nelson and Drought, 1992; Parise and Meers, 1986; Plowles, 1973; Pollard, 1991; Ratcliff, 1989; Relman, 1980; Rice, 1988; Schel, 1989; Scofield, 1991; Somerville, 1993; Turner, 1987; Weigold, 1985; Wiernik, 1982; Wolf, 1991; Zola, 1979; 1980).

8 Rawlinson (1987:373) articulates this Foucaultian notion of biomedical science as but one 'way' of knowing when he writes that 'a genealogical analysis of modern scientific medicine reveals that the epistemological and political knowledge and power, are ineluctably intertwined, so that truth is not so much discovered - as if it lay ready-made in objective reality patiently awaiting the articulate voice of science - as produced according to regular and identifiable procedures that determine in any given historical situation what it is possible to say, who is authorized to speak, what can become an object of scientific inquiry, and how knowledge is to be tested, accumulated, and dispersed.'

9 Such institutional care will refer to tertiary hospital care where statistics indicate the majority of people in our society die.

10 As Kohut and Kohut (1984:8) point out, there is a continuum from hospital based care to community based hospice care.

2 The postmodern lens

> The Hungarian Nobel laureate, Albert Szent-Gyorgi, once said that 'Research is to see what everyone else has seen and to think what no one else has thought' (Lamers, 1988).

This chapter will begin to articulate the epistemological assumptions which underpin the postmodern approach to this study. Because postmodern theorising does not lend itself to any foundational assumptions, the ideas presented in the following discussion will reflect my own particular construction of postmodern notions which are considered essential to understanding the process of engaging in this research.

Postmodernism has been chosen because of the attractiveness and usefulness of the ideas generated by such epistemological and metaphysical perspectives. In particular, the notion of discourse, the relationship of discourse to power, a respect for a multiplicity of voices, the honesty and humility encouraged by ideas of self-reflexivity, and a searching critical orientation which challenges the possibility of arriving at ultimate truth or shared foundational values, are some of the important features of the postmodern approach which I have found to be useful.

This discussion begins by articulating the positivist, scientific notions of neutrality, objectivity and truth which frame the dominant 'way' western technologised society understands and consequently (as will be shown in later chapters) responds to, issues of death and dying. It will be argued that these modernist epistemological assumptions translate into a reductionist physiological understanding of death (the biomedical model), which disguised as truth are in a direct relationship to the construction of reality for the dying. The metaphor for this reality is 'body as machine', not individual as spiritual entity.

The aim of this discussion will be to move from such restricted scientific understandings to a different 'way' of doing research based on a postmodern approach. Such an approach emphasises heterogeneity and a multiplicity of ways of seeing. Modernist absolute claims to rational truth are replaced by notions of discourse, power, and researcher subjectivity. The Enlightenment's belief in rationalism is replaced by an understanding of power and resistance both through and within discourse.

Based on this different 'way' of approaching this topic, a focus on discourse and the ideas associated with deconstruction will be highlighted as notions central to engaging in this research. The hope and expectation is that such an alternative research direction will make a modest contribution to including in our body of research on dying, ideas marginalised by more conservative research methodologies. In particular, it will be argued (and demonstrated later in this work), such a postmodern approach allows the inclusion of the notion of spirituality which is not easily accommodated by modernist research methodologies.

The scientific 'way' of seeing

> Different discourses (as opposed to theories) about the world are assessed not in terms of their truth, i.e., accuracy of representation, but rather as different ways of talking about the world (Mumby, 1988:130).

The starting point for this discussion is an acknowledgment that the 'way' our society responds to those who are dying is predominantly through the biomedical approach (Lather, 1991:105; Cassell, 1991a:x) and that such positivist, scientific understandings are limited when exploring questions about death and dying. A postmodern approach, it will be suggested, provides insights which lead to thinking differently about these issues. To understand this difference, it is important to first explore the notions involved in biomedicine.

The modernist scientific beliefs which underpin our medical interventions are based on positivist, scientific notions of neutrality and objectivity (Capra, 1990; Oldroyd, 1986; Fay, 1975). Methodologically, the researcher is somehow situated outside of 'reality', looking in, observing, recording and analysing in a vacuum of neutrality, untainted by life experience, personal values, culture, or history. Capra refers to this phenomenon as a 'guarantee (of) scientific objectivity by eliminating any reference to the observer' (1990:416). The 'facts' gathered by such a method are prized and valued because of the very process of achieving neutrality by strict methodological processes. Methodological strictness is seen to ensure objectivity and the production of truth (Chalmers, 1976:1). Issues such as the social power behind whoever commissions the research, the ideological and philosophical perspectives of those who couch the research questions, the interests of those who fund the research, and reasons why such research was considered important in the first place, are not seen as impacting on or detracting from the absoluteness of the 'truth' produced. As long as the method is strict and legitimated as an approved way of researching, 'truth' is claimed. [1]

Such an orientation to manufacturing 'truth' through research is based on a linear, teleological rationality (Lather, 1991:105). The modernist scientific project is based on the assumption that the accumulation of such 'facts' will lead to progress by providing the positive power through understanding to control and improve the human condition. Through a linear rationality, progress is intricately tied to the accumulation of knowledge inscribed as objective truth (Fox, 1991:722; Plowles, 1973).[2] Questions of values, and ontological considerations about what it is to be human, (not only now but in the future) are suppressed in a way of knowing that assumes a shared teleological view of human progress.

In a rationality that leads from the assumed production of truth to a perceived shared teleological understanding of human progress and control of human destiny, such a world view eliminates by denial, the possibility that it could be but one value position and discourse among many possibilities. The probability that such a notion of neutrality may itself only be the reflection of a western scientific academic tradition is avoided in an epistemology which suppresses such questions by its insistence on the fact that objectivity *is* the method.[3] Reified to truth, rather than accepted as but one value laden way of seeing, the scientific method has a powerful influence over the social construction of knowledge.

Foucault writes extensively on this link between the production of truth and issues of power. Importantly, for this discussion on the scientific method, he states, 'truth isn't outside power, or lacking in power...(T)ruth is a thing of this world: it is produced only by virtue of multiple forms of constraint. And it induces regular effects of power. Each society has its regime of truth, its 'general politics' of truth; that is, the types of discourse which it accepts and makes function as true; the mechanisms and instances which enable one to distinguish true and false statements, the means by which each is sanctioned; the techniques and procedures accorded value in the acquisition of truth; the status of those who are charged with saying what counts as true' (Foucault in Rabinow, 1984:73). The scientific method is seen as one such regime of truth.

This has particular relevance to the topic of dying, (explored in detail in Chapter 7), where the questions asked, what is legitimated to be fact, what issues are funded for research, and which directions are seen to be important for future progress, are all determined by funding bodies espousing the scientific method. In short, such a positivist, scientific way of knowing is in a direct relationship with 'truth' production, and hence, the creation and inscription of what is deemed to be 'reality'.

As will be discussed later in this work (Chapter 8), this rational, positivistic, scientific approach when focused on issues of death and dying translates into a reductionist, physiological understanding.[4] Progress is seen to be achieved by an engineering approach to medicine (Plowles, 1973), which seeks to eliminate the enemy of death.[5] The body becomes a machine to be understood physically, worked on mechanically, and made to last as long as possible (Capra, 1990). The challenge is seen to be discovering the cure to disease (Hart, 1985:10) in an ongoing 'battle' against death.

The postmodern challenge

> Simplifying to the extreme, I define *postmodern* as incredulity toward metanarratives (Lyotard, 1984:xxiv).

Lyotard's work, 'The Postmodern Condition' (1984), the *locus classicus* of the postmodern era, argues against the credibility of the legitimation of overarching philosophies of history, such as the Enlightenment story of science (Fraser and Nicholson, 1988:376). The teleological rationality of science, predicated on notions of objective truth, is seen as but one Grand Theory among many other claims to totalising knowledge. Rather than viewing the understandings arising from science as truth, a postmodern *episteme* situates such knowledge historically, culturally and philosophically as an expression of modernist ways of seeing the world. A postmodern approach views the scientific method as an expression of the 'Age of Enlightenment' and the 'Scientific Revolution', rather than any absolute or foundational claim to truth.[6] The postmodern model of science challenges such notions of 'truth' as but one metanarrative. The postmodern approach is to view all grand theories as totalising systems, which try to synthesise, or more correctly impose, a construction of reality from one view point.[7] Thus, a postmodern respect for heterogeneity and a multiplicity of ways of seeing rejects all such systems of totalising thought (Docherty, 1990:213).

This then questions the possibility of one rationality which can speak for all,[8] and replaces it with a fragmented, diversified and decentralising way of speaking about the construction of reality (Turner, 1990:16). Consequently, claims to universality, progress and autonomy in science are no longer seen as absolute truths but rather as myths which are now debunked (Lather, 1991:13).[9]

Rather than seek absolute claims to theoretical truth, the postmodern concern is with exploring the limits of speculative reason, acknowledging as important the irreducible problems in any epistemological assumptions about the notion of truth (Norris, 1989:221; Smyth, 1991:114). Best and Kellner sum up the postmodern epistemological position as an acknowledgment that, 'knowledge is perspectival in nature, requiring multiple viewpoints to interpret a heterogeneous reality' (1991:35).

The idea of grand theory in postmodern thought becomes replaced by the notion of discourse. A postmodern interpretative framework understands the scientific method as but one, although admittedly a first-order discourse, among many other discourses (Fraser and Nicholson, 1988:377).

Rather than being situated within the positivist enlightenment story, postmodern writers begin to explore the very notions signified by such words as science, reason, enlightenment and humanity. There is a heightened awareness that these words are but conceptual signposts, that do not exist in the nature of things but, as with all our language, reflect our philosophical systems (Dear, 1988). Postmodern analysis emphasises that no knowledge can be assessed outside the context of the meaning endowed and made possible by such social systems as culture, tradition, and language games (Bauman,

1988:226).

The postmodern concern is to fracture, explore difference, and affirm a multiplicity of epistemological viewpoints.[10] Any construction and interpretation of reality is built on an appreciation of the fallibility of that particular point of view. The historical, cultural, and sociological influences on the producers of theory are considered as important as the very theories they produce.[11] Absolute claims to truth are replaced by an understanding of knowledge which is tentative, probabilistic, and revisable in principle (Kellner, 1988:251).

According to a postmodern approach, then, claims of truth are displaced by understandings of discourse. One important consequence of the use of this very useful notion of discourse, which will be demonstrated throughout this research is that it allows the exploration of ideas such as spirituality, which are marginalised and omitted from the biomedical discourse.

Discourse on discourse

To reiterate, a postmodern approach rejects the grand narrative, whether it be about science, the enlightenment, humanity or progressive medicine (Fox, 1991; Fraser and Nicholson, 1988; Lather, 1991; Turner, 1990). All forms of totalising thought are deemed epistemologically fragile, as is the belief in an archimedean spot which could function as a lever to ultimate truth (Fox, 1991:711). Thus, this research wishes to explore notions of discourse rather than to make absolute claims to truth.

The notion of discourse is difficult to define for two reasons. Firstly, most postmodern writers seem to make the implicit assumption that the notion of discourse is understood and this meaning is shared by the reader. There are few attempts at clarifying the notion' [12] (although it is used extensively), and where attempts are made there is no definitional agreement (Davies, 1994:1; Fairclough, 1989:24; Fairclough, 1992:3; Lather, 1991:vii; Weedon, 1987:108). Secondly, this definitional uncertainty embraces a multiplicity of implied meanings. Even within this research, the notion of discourse will vary depending on the context of the discussion. Both the Foucaultian theoretical notion of discourse (Weedon, 1987:108), and Fairclough's social practice notions (Fairclough, 1992:64), will be referred to throughout this work as useful ideas for developing insights. It is important then, to set the stage for later discussions to introduce and explore these two compatible but different notions of discourse.

The Foucaultian notion of discourse

The Foucaultian notion of discourse is very theoretical and refers to the different ways of structuring areas of knowledge and social practice (Fairclough, 1992:3). Foucault's work (1972) traces such 'knowledges' or discourses historically to show how they have developed over time, through a process known as the 'archaeology' of knowledge.

Significantly, for the present discussion, one such archaeological investigation was a study of the development of biomedicine (Foucault, 1973). As will be examined in a later chapter, (Chapter 8), the reductionist, physiological, medically directed focus of such a medical discourse is described by Foucault as the 'clinical gaze' (1973:120).

The fundamental concern of the Foucaultian notion of discourse is the way in which one particular statement appears rather than another in any specific socio-historical context (Davies, 1994:1). Why, for example, do we predominantly refer to those who are dying as patients and couch their dying trajectory in clinical terms? Why is the word spiritual omitted from textbooks which educate physicians about how to work with the terminally ill? Why are we as a society so comfortable with terms such as the 'battle' against death or the 'war' against cancer? Why has the word holism only recently appeared in our health vocabulary?

These words, according to notions of discourse, do not randomly and arbitrarily appear, but rather are situated in the innumerable discourses running through our society. Such discourses are historically, culturally and socially constructed. Discourses are seen by postmodern theorists as the site where different social groups struggle for hegemony, and hence the opportunity to impose through the language of discourse their own production of meaning and ideology (Best and Kellner, 1991:26).

Foucault was interested in how the subject was socially and historically constructed through related discourses (Davies, 1994:1), whereby the individual is seen as the node or post where simultaneously a number of distinct discourses will converge with varying degrees of effectivity (Valverde, 1991:182). Both domination by, and resistance to, such hegemonic discourses coexist at all societal levels and at any point in time.

By incorporating all these ideas of knowledge, power and subjectivity, Weedon defines the Foucaultian theoretical notion of discourse as 'ways of constituting knowledge, together with the social practices, forms of subjectivity and power relations which inhere in such knowledges and the relations between them' (1987:108). Such a Foucaultian understanding of the notion of discourse will be used when referring to the important discourses seen to be running through Karuna Hospice Service, which include the bio-medical discourse, the hospice discourse, the spiritual discourse and the Buddhist discourse.

Discourse as 'actual talk'

Alternatively, discourse can be interpreted in more pragmatic, local, contextual terms as the actual words or 'talk' of individuals in their day to day experience, as seen by the following definition by Kress (cited in Davies, 1994:17). He defines discourse as,

> systematically organised ways of talking .. systematically-organised sets of

statements which give expression to the meanings and values of an institution. Beyond that, they define, describe and delimit what it is possible to say and not possible to say (and by extension - what it is possible to do or not to do) with respect to the area of concern of that institution, whether marginally or centrally. A discourse provides a set of possible statements about a given area, and organises and gives structure to the manner in which a particular topic, object, process is to be talked about. In that it provides descriptions, rules, permissions and prohibitions of social and individual action.

Such a notion of discourse will be used when referring to the every day discursive practices of KHS. This interpretation of the term discourse refers to the 'actual talk or writing' (Fairclough, 1989:29) of those associated with KHS and this will form the basis for the collection of the language/texts, (as will be discussed in later chapters).

Such 'talk' reflects not only the limits and possibilities of KHS's meaning-making and values, but also incorporates the impact of the more powerful, historically constituted social discourses. When examining such localised examples of discourse, the powerful, historically determined discourses (such as biomedicine and Buddhism) will be emphasised. In terms of these two compatible and interrelated, yet different definitions of discourse, it is therefore possible within this research to speak of the contradiction of the many discourses within KHS's discourse.

Discourse and power - the important link

In the literature on the postmodern approach, as has already been indicated, discourse and power are intrinsically linked (Smyth, 1991:112). This theme of the close association of power and discourse will be developed throughout this work. It will suffice, however, in this introductory chapter to simply set the stage by articulating some of the initial important notions associated with discourse and power that will be expanded upon throughout the analysis. Such notions challenge the modernist idea of rationality by an understanding that recognises the 'will to power' in all discourses.

The modernist project of enlightenment, it has already been explained, was based on a belief in the possibility and value of rationalism. This ethos of balanced consideration and objective analysis resonated with great force through our dominant discourses such as science, medicine and ethics (McGrath, 1994:152). Certainly the hallmark of the era of modernity was the certainty, the superiority and self-confidence promised by the 'progressive' values of rationality (Bauman, 1988:220).

As will be demonstrated by the following discussion many postmodern writers have contributed insights which suggest that the very idea of rationality is an illusion. A postmodern epistemology challenges the notions underpinning the language of reason: the present suspicion being that 'there is no reason, only reasons' (Featherstone, 1988:209).

The postmodern approach builds on Nietzsche's notion that the will to truth and knowledge is indistinguishable from the 'will to power'. Foucault challenges the belief in the rationality of the Enlightenment by linking the production of knowledge through discourse with power (Best and Kellner, 1991:34-5). All discourses, according to Foucault (1980:101), are produced by power.[13] Equally, power is constituted through discourse by, as Fox explains (1991:723), the creation and imposition through 'talk' of a 'locally produced knowledgeability about the world and its inhabitants'. In short, discourses provide the signs and symbols, the concepts and the meaning through which a version of reality is both produced and legitimated. The postmodern era embraces this Foucaultian notion of power/knowledge with its suspicion that the production of knowledge and the construction of reality through discourse is a political, not rational process.

Power, according to Foucault, is omnipresent; it is the societal force behind discourse as well as constantly being produced through and within discourses (Van Dijk, 1989:22). To take an example relevant to this work, medicocentric power inherent in the biomedical discourse dominates our society's response to death and dying.[14] Such power determines who cares for the dying, where people die, what issues are considered important in understanding the dying process, which professionals are in control of the decision-making and the options offered to those who are dying.[15]

Although discursive power is interpreted as omnipresent, this does not negate the possibility of resistance. This question of resistance, however, is a contentious issue of debate in the postmodern literature, with different authors providing varying insight and conclusions on the matter. Foucault's work, for example, stresses the enormous power of discourse to dominate and limit the individual (1980; 1986). Authors such as Fox (1993:27), however, engage in a critique of such omnipresent power and hence suggest the possibility of retaining some space for creativity and the opportunity for resistance. For Fox (1993:57) resistance is both ubiquitous and unexceptional. Similarly, Lyotard offers the optimistic message that 'no one, not even the least privileged among us, is ever entirely powerless over the messages that traverse and position him at the post of sender, addressee, or referent' (1984:15). Such optimism will be taken as a starting point for this work. In short, the approach to power will be that whilst discourse is constitutive of the talk and hence the action of individuals, at the same time, some discursive space is allowed for creativity in the interpretation of such messages and the opportunity for some degree of resistance.

The emphasis throughout this discussion of discourse and power, it should be noted, is that the medium for the social connection is language. The social relations of power are produced, maintained, negotiated and changed through the vehicle of language (Fairclough, 1989:1). The postmodern concern with discourse is, indeed, a concern with 'talk'.This suggests that discursive practices are an important medium through which an understanding can be developed of how social relations are produced and reproduced.

Day-to-day discursive processes materially 'fix' ideological meaning and hence affirm conceptions of reality. According to Mumby and Stohl, 'social collectives come to privilege certain articulations of reality over others' (1991:313). For example, the 'talk' of KHS will be constitutive of one such reality. KHS will be seen as being in an active relationship to the construction of reality; such constructions will be through and within the discourses impacting on, and generated by, this organisation over time. An examination of the 'talk' of KHS will thus be seen as the medium for understanding the complexity and interrelationship of significant discourses relevant to this organisation, and will also provide insights into the social relationships of power.

Of central importance to understanding such a postmodern approach to power/knowledge is the notion that reality is defined as much by what is not spoken, as by concepts that are. Power is maintained by concepts silenced, ideas not affirmed ('signified absence') (Mumby and Stohl, 1991), as much as by the construction of meaning through words used. Interpreted as such, power is a process, a double discourse which constantly disavows and then reinscripts control (Smyth, 1991:113).

Such theoretical conceptualisation defines power from within discursive practices, rather than *over* organisational members: 'discourse, as both the medium and outcome of this construction process, simultaneously negates and affirms different conceptual and experiential possibilities' (Mumby and Stohl, 1991:319).

Hence, the postmodern concern is with how power is constituted through discourses (Fox, 1991:723). As will be seen by the following discussion, the 'givenness' of privileged discourses are explored to disclose the concealed power and self-interest (Aronowitz, 1992:55). Postmodernist interpretative frames embrace the Foucaultian shift from paradigm to discourse, from an ontological belief in truth of progress, to a discourse on discourse.

Developing insights based on notions of deconstruction

The idea of discourse has so far been described as a notion central to this research. The question then arises as to how to explore such notions of discourse whilst engaging in research?

One process of analysing discourse is through the 'activity' of deconstruction. 'Deconstruction is the dismantling of conceptual oppositions, the taking apart of hierarchical systems of thought which can then be reinscribed within a different order of textual signification' (Norris, 1987:19). Our concepts, ideas and thoughts are embedded in language, which in turn is constrained by conscious and unconscious strategies of exclusion and repression, hiding to varying degrees, contradictions and paradoxes. Deconstruction is an activity aimed at exposing these contradictions and paradoxes (Dear, 1988), whereby the deconstructed centre is replaced by the freeplay of discursive expression (Lemert, 1992:31). Derrida's process of deconstruction is based on an understanding of the creation of meaning through a system of pairs which signify opposites. Such binary opposites, as represented in the following 'deconstruction graphics' (Elam, 1994:11) eg.

mind/body, subject/object, male/female, create the illusion of stability through the privileging of one term in the pair over the opposite. 'Deconstruction is therefore the operation through which these oppositions can be at least partially undermined, and alternative readings made possible' (Mumby and Stohl, 1991:318).

Deconstruction is not an event, but an ongoing process of analysis that challenges dogma. The goal of deconstruction is to challenge, to play with ideas, to demystify, to disrupt the comforting exclusiveness of our thought (Lather, 1991:13); it is not to achieve theoretical wholeness nor a dialectical resolution. Characterising the fluidity of postmodern intellectual activity, deconstruction never ends (Fox, 1991: 742).

Although it is claimed that deconstruction is a process, an activity of reading rather than an irreducibly defined method or concept (Norris, 1982:1; Norris, 1987:27; Smart, 1993:13), there is evidence within the literature on postmodernism of its use in research for examining organisational discourse (Cheek and Rudge, 1994; Mumby and Stohl, 1991). Such deconstruction is concerned not only with how signification legitimates the sectional interests of hegemonic groups, but most importantly, with how an illumination of the 'signified absence', (the implicit but unspoken concepts), contributes to an understanding of the process of resistance and control in relation to hegemonic groups. Is it in Karuna's interests to privilege, and hence silence the same concepts as the hegemonic, biomedical discourse? Are there ideas expressed in Karuna's discourse which would in any way challenge (or accommodate) the power and control of technologised medicine?

These ideas developed by writers who use the process of deconstruction are considered both useful and relevant for developing this analysis. Throughout the process of engaging in the interpretation of data such notions will inform the analysis. The emphasis here is on the usefulness of the ideas rather than any explicit idea of a research process.

Although any adherence to a well defined process used by writers who use deconstruction is rejected for this work, it is considered of benefit to explore descriptions of deconstruction in an attempt to further clarify the ideas which will be used. According to Smart, deconstruction can be broken down into a three step process (1993:13). Firstly, the binary concepts used in the organisational discourse need to be identified. As will be discussed later in this work, one such example of a binary concept surfacing in the discourse of KHS is that of alternative/mainstream implying a nonconforming (KHS) /conservative (mainstream health professionals) binary opposite value base. Secondly, once isolated, the dependent terms need to be replaced by a positive term. To continue the example, the 'will to serve', to help and to care are seen as positive values shared by both positions. Thirdly, a transcendent expression, which is both and neither of the terms, needs to be conceptualised. To complete the example, the notion of an 'exemplary counter institution' (Starr, 1979:246), is used as a concept that voiced the silenced notions of conservatism in KHS's alternative discourse. Such insights from the writers of deconstruction, show KHS's discourse to be not necessarily the binary opposite of mainstream professional discourse, but rather similar in many aspects.

However, such an understanding of the ideas underpinning deconstruction, for the purposes of this work, seems particularly mechanistic and defined. The use of ideas from writers who engage in deconstruction will be a far more intuitive process, based on moments of insights which cannot be translated into such a logical, sequential, orderly process. Although Smart's definition is helpful in understanding the rationale for the deconstructive process, it has a positivistic flavour of inscribing a rigid description[16] which detracts from the postmodern orientation towards a conceptual openness of playing with ideas. Whilst acknowledging the usefulness of such a description, this work is situated in Elam's notion (1994:4-5), of allowing the 'isness' of the authors use of ideas associated with the deconstructive reading of texts, to unfold through the actual doing of the research. This position accepts that a universally agreed upon definition of deconstruction is 'highly undesirable' because of its potential to lead to 'caricature, dismissal, and unnecessary limits' placed on thought (ibid).

The experience of deconstructive thinking during the work on this research resembled less the sequential stages defined above, and more Norris's description (1989:216) of *mise en abyme,* the moments of infinite regression, which reveals the non-existence of ultimate ground. To finish with the example given, it was a moment of insight and considerable surprise, rather than one of logical analysis, to arrive at the deconstructive conclusion that there were major conservative elements in the discourse of what was originally believed to be a very alternative organisation. In retrospect, Norris's *mise en abyme* seems to be closer to a description of the process than Smart's three step logical sequence.

Underpinning such an interpretation was a concern to illuminate the basic Foucaultian questions, as articulated by Barrett (1991:126), which ask - According to what rules has a particular statement been made? According to what rules could other similar statements be made? How is it that one particular statement appeared rather than another? In relation to Karuna Hospice Service, such questions will seek insights not only into the working of this organisation but also into the relationship of its discourse with the 'first order' discourse of the biomedical model.

Thus, the use of notions associated with deconstruction will inform a playful reading of the language/texts gathered for this research. Such an engagement in interpreting data need not come up with conclusive answers to problems posed but, as explained before, may be a useful medium for developing research questions.

The researcher's 'will to power'

How we speak and write tells us more about our own inscribed selves, about the way that language writes us, than about the 'object' of our gaze. The trick is to see the will to power in our work as clearly as we see the will to truth. (Smart, 1993:119).

The subjectivity of the author, or producer of knowledge, is now viewed as an integral factor to the understanding of any text (research for the purpose of this paper is taken to be a text). This epistemic suspicion that discourses cannot escape the mark of their producers, as defined by their socio/historical embeddedness, identity and interests, is the core of the postmodern approach (Seidman, 1992:68).

In the postmodern approach to research, issues of research integrity move from notions of maintaining objectivity and eliminating bias, to concerns with articulating the researcher's individual 'will to power', and demonstrating commitment to self-reflexivity throughout the research process. As will be seen by the detailed discussion of Chapter 3, the influence of the researcher will be seen as important in exploring the research process as the characteristics of the research participants. Emphasis is placed on the motivation, background, attitudes and philosophy of the researcher, which are documented as important factors in the construction of the research outcome. Ultimately, all research is open to the reading of others, in which notions silenced can be explored to provide further insights into the conclusions reached. The responsibility for authorship of this research is acknowledged, and the possibility of alternative readings accepted.

An important assumption for this work is a rejection of the 'subject/object separation', which argues for validity and objectivity in maintaining a strict separation between researcher and research subject (McCarl Nielsen, 1990:76; Weedon, 1987:7). As such, the theoretical validity of this work cannot be judged by a fixed or pre-given form. As Gunew explains, such postmodern research must be understood by its 'intersubjective effects, that is, its capacity to be shared, understood, and communicated by those occupying similar positions: and also by its intertextual effects, that is, its capacity to affirm or undermine various prevailing or subordinate discursive systems, and the effects it has on other discourses' (1990:168). In particular, this study will be situated within (and hence shared, understood and communicated to others engaged in) the discourses on hospice/palliative care, bioethics and spirituality.

Postmodern irony

Central to this research is an epistemological, some would say political, tension between accepting as an expression of their reality what people in a local, concrete setting learn to say about their conditions, acknowledging that reality, and yet, analysing such statements within a theoretical framework which sees reality as figurative, inescapably embedded in language, which is socio/historically situated. Such research is engaged in the paradox of questioning reality while simultaneously writing about reality: presenting research insights through the medium of language while accepting that language is provisional not final.

Postmodern writers accept this challenge through the idea of irony. They accept this tension and are prepared to make statements while at the same time they recognise that they cannot be finally persuasive against other such statements (Lemert, 1992:20). Rorty describes ironists as 'never quite able to take themselves seriously because (they are) always aware that the terms in which they describe themselves are subject to change, always aware of the contingency and fragility of their final vocabularies, and thus of their selves' (1989:73-4).

Anticipating, acknowledging and responding to criticisms of the postmodern approach

So far then, an outline has been given of the contribution of relevant postmodern ideas. Particular emphasis has been placed on the examination of the research texts through the literature on discourse and the insights of deconstruction. The challenge, it has been argued, is to move from secular, modernist, scientific understandings of end-of-life issues to the 'yet to be fully explored' postmodern approach.

A vital part of accepting that challenge, however, is to acknowledge the problems and concerns which arise from such theorising. It will be the task of the last part of this chapter to begin to explore such conceptual concerns.

Although an enormous amount of literature has now been written and accepted across many disciplines on postmodern epistemological ideas, such notions are (in comparison to the three hundred year old history of entrenched modernist concepts) relatively new and innovative. As with all creative adventures, a sojourn into this newly emerging field entails some risk: in this case it is the sacrificing of the comfort and certainty of the known[17] for the intellectual satisfaction and sense of personal integrity associated with exploring ideas in the hope of making a positive contribution.

The inescapable choice

> But now I have come to believe that the whole world is an enigma, a harmless enigma that is made terrible by our own mad attempt to interpret it as though it had an underlying truth (Eco, 1989:95).

Such epistemological risk taking has not been a deliberated intellectual choice but rather the inevitable outcome of ruminating on a number of concerns. These concerns evolved from direct and extensive experience with the dehumanising impact of the biomedical model on the experience of dying. My ongoing involvement in oncology and palliative care through my previous postgraduate work on chemotherapy continually affirms and reinscribes the seriousness of the problems of biomedicine in this regard.

Paralleling these ongoing concerns is my sense of the fragility of all understanding and my profound concern with the limits and potential danger of absolute knowing. This journey into the evolving field of postmodern research has, consequently, seemed like a vital imperative necessary to maintain intellectual integrity rather than a calculated intellectual option. To undertake the completion of this research requires an enormous commitment of time and energy, which would not (to my mind) have been justified if the integrity born of intellectual curiosity was sacrificed for the safety of a more easily legitimated methodology.

There are, it will be argued, three 'key' notions, (as outlined in the previous discussion), which make a commitment to an exploration of postmodernism for this research, in the mind of this writer, not a choice but an inescapable direction. A summary of these notions is important for situating, and understanding, the response to criticisms of postmodernism as will be outlined in the following discussion.

These notions include, firstly, the important question of the unavoidable heterogeneity: the complex, arguably incommensurable , unalterable plurality of the many metaphysical and epistemological 'realities' of the present postmodern world.[18] At the price of uncertainty, an understanding of the postmodern notion of relativism begins to confront such a groundless heterogeneity, which is so important for any research with a focus on questions of bioethics and death-and-dying.

Secondly, this work is concerned with unquantifiable, perhaps indefinable, indescribable and unknowable, esoteric notions of spirituality, meaning making and holism, which as later discussions will show, are presently excluded from 'mainstream' research. Postmodern notions of discourse, most importantly, provide the 'vehicle', where at least these ideas become discussable. Captured as discourse, examined as discursive practices that translate into subjectivities, there is not the onus on the researcher to 'prove' or 'disprove' the existence or otherwise of such expressed realities. A postmodern approach, thus, importantly, opens research possibilities for those interested in the less quantifiable dimension of existence. It opens the possibility, for those interested, of translating issues of transcendental reality, into a 'do-able' research project.

Thirdly, and lastly, the anti-foundational orientation to truth and value, which positions all statements within the subjectivity of language, history and culture (to name but a few variables), once acknowledged, permeates all epistemological and metaphysical understandings. Comforting as it must have been to operate from an absolutist, or dogmatic position, for this author this appears to no longer be an option. Although criticism of the postmodern approach will be acknowledged and explored, there seems at present to be no escaping such a relativistic position.

These three factors of heterogeneity, anti-positivism and anti-foundationalism (or relativism), not only make postmodernism attractive, but inescapable. Consequently, the 'will to power' underpinning this text, is an inescapable philosophical commitment to an exploration of postmodern ideas. Criticisms, thus, will be viewed and presented as firstly, modernist misinterpretations of postmodern understanding, or secondly, understandable angst over difficult to accept recent direction in epistemology, or thirdly, as yet to be resolved paradoxes, or contradictions in an emergent area of theorising. Criticism is seen as inevitable, towards an epistemology that challenges entrenched modernist ways of thinking.[19] Such criticism is an important source of questions: some to be responded to and resolved, others to lead to further questioning. These questions will be addressed, with a will to avoid inscribing certainty and closure.

Although this journey into postmodern research is defended as an inevitable result of the author's intellectual 'will to power' this does not necessarily imply that (particularly at this early stage of the exploration of these ideas) such postmodern notion will not have problems. It is acknowledged that such a 'postmodern lens' is far from unproblematic. The point of this research is to begin to explore such ideas, to take up the challenge of looking in new directions: in short, to contribute rather than master.

Notions raised in this discussion will be extended and explored, both through the 'doing of the research', and by a concluding chapter of reflection on the value and contribution of postmodernism to bioethics and research. An important caveat to the following discussion, however, is that whilst acknowledging the diversity of writings that are lumped together under the title of postmodernism (Kellner, 1988:241),this discussion can only respond to criticisms of the interpretation of the term as inscribed in this research.[20]

This discussion will move from an exploration of the broader criticisms of the vexed question of the demise of the grand narrative and the endless relativism such an epistemological vacuum implies, to a focus on the detailed critiques of postmodern ideas associated with deconstruction.

A beginning to the discussion then, will be the concerns about relativism. Situated in an awareness that notions of postmodernism are as yet, 'undertheorized' (Kellner, 1988:241), it is again emphasised that this discussion wishes to raise, acknowledge and make some contribution to understanding, but not necessarily resolve, such problematics.

The question of relativism

> There are limits to the power of reason such that it is a mistake to speak of '*the* truth'. There is no single and final truth about ourselves which can definitively reveal who we are and what we ought to become. *This is difficult to accept* (Fay, 1987:206; Author's emphasis).

Although, it is now taken as a given that no knowledge can be validated outside the context of culture, tradition and language, the epistemological relativism such a notion suggests, creates considerable academic, ideological angst. The fear seems to be that if our accepted ideas on science and knowing are challenged, then the very foundation for saying anything is lost (Lather, 1991:xi).[21]

This postmodern research does not seek to problematise as nihilist, the multiplicity of voices characteristic of relativism. Rather than mourn the loss of clarity and security of foundationalism,[22] this work embraces with enthusiasm Lyotard's notion of the 'replacement of narrative knowledge by a plurality of language games, and universalism by localism' (Featherstone, 1988:198). Such plurality and localism, with its concomitant lack of apology for grand theory is, it is argued, *the* valued ingredient of this postmodern approach to research.[23] As Lather, when similarly responding to such criticism explains,

> Rather than as 'crisis' such questioning of basic assumptions might be seen as an effort to break out of the limitations of increasingly inadequate category systems and toward theory capable of grasping the complexities of people and cultures they create - theories outside of binary logics of certainty, non-contradiction, totality and linearity (1991:xvi).

The antifoundational perspectives of postmodernism do, indeed, sacrifice a sense of absolute and certain knowing, the comforting closure of linear rationality and the teleological optimism of definite and finite solutions.[24] Such relativism (although implied by critics of the postmodern approach as a criticism) is welcome in this work, as a liberating statement of the inevitable and obvious.[25] As Bauman, states the case, 'there are *many* "life-worlds", *many* "language-games". No external point of view is conceivable to reduce this variety' (1988:229).

The ideological angst in relation to relativism, it is argued, must be deeper than a denial of the inevitable and obvious: deeper than some detached fantasising about the possibility of an homogeneous and certain world of grand theory. Perhaps Harding is closer to decentring the fear of relativism when she writes,

> Historically, relativism appears as an intellectual possibility, and as a 'problem', only for dominating groups at the point where the hegemony of their views is being challenged (1987:115).

The very resistance to postmodern ideas, according to Norris (1985:18) is indicative of its 'salutary power to disturb'. If this is the basis of the fear, than it is an appropriate basis, because as noted by Smyth (1991:114), one of the aims of postmodernism is 'to interrogate and demystify totalising systems that unify with an eye to power'.

Behind this modernist fear of losing control, is the association of relativism with irrationality, or the Nietzschean anger of nihilism. Postmodernism can, has and will be used for nihilist reasons. This is acknowledged, but only as part of the story. That a postmodern outlook, and particularly one that incorporates ideas of deconstruction, recognises that there can never be certainty (that the 'right' questions are asked or the 'correct' answers given) does not mean, *ipso facto,* that such an epistemology is invariably condemned to relativistic nihilism or political inaction (Elam, 1994:31). The challenge is to maintain the courage to think and act within an uncertain framework (Lather, 1991:13). That this is possible is evidenced by the notion that authors who embrace the postmodern, can and do, situate themselves in a range of positions, including, for example, a critical framework (Elam, 1994; Foster, 1985; Huyssen, 1987:xvi; Lather, 1991:1), feminism, (Elam, 1994; Fraser and Nicholson, 1988; Lather, 1991; Weedon, 1987), and ecology, (Gare, 1995).

Humility, openness and an epistemic suspicion that any discussion of the human condition must include 'complex incommensurable teleologies, of heterogeneity in social, society and aesthetic experience' (Featherstone, 1988:209), is interpreted, for the purposes of this work, positively rather than as a criticism. Postmodern relativism gives permission to let go of the Cartesian-Lockean-Kantian tradition of an absolute and detached knowing, creating the opportunity to move from a modernist reliance on metanarratives, to an epistemic opportunity which 'refines our sensitivity to differences and reinforces our ability to tolerate the incommensurable' (Lyotard, 1984:xxv). Such uncertainty and undecidability need not translate into nihilistic relativism, and inaction, but a politics that prizes difference and the responsibility to decide. [26] To decide not to act, is an act of decision. There is no escaping the existential responsibility of decision making.[27]

Whether viewing relativism as problematic or liberating, it appears to the author that there is no escaping such plurality of thought. As Norris argues, we have reached a point of no return -

> From the assumption that all truths are 'relative to language' it is strictly impossible *not* to arrive at some form of wholesale epistemological scepticism. Only a theory that reverses that assumption - and offers good grounds for so doing - can hope to turn back the more unwelcome effects of this widespread relativist drift (985:217).

The vexed question of the grand narrative

Underpinning this concern about postmodern relativism, is the question of whether grand theory is 'To Be? Or not to Be?'. As has been discussed in detail earlier in the chapter, the postmodern approach is built around a deep suspicion of the claims to truth of any totalising system of theory. Such a question is both vexed and ongoing, with theorising responses ranging from a rejection of grand theory, *tout court* (Lyotard, 1984), to a serious exploration of the possibility of developing a postmodern grand theory (Gare, 1995).[28]

The epistemological position of this work approximates Jameson's suggestion (Lyotard, 1984:xii), that perhaps we are condemned to narratives, as an indispensable part of social theorising. The danger lies not so much in the narrative, but in the grand theory, for as Elam explains, 'any attempt to describe society exhaustively runs the risk of totalitarianism' (1994:105). This research whilst situated in the rejection of the metanarrative, would also privilege the tension, the contradiction, the paradox, of the possible usefulness of the partial, probabilistic, fallible role of the very grand theory it marginalises. Lather expresses this position well when she writes,

> To write 'postmodern' is to simultaneously use and call into question a discourse, to both challenge and inscribe dominant meaning systems in ways that construct our own categories and frameworks as contingent, positioned, partial (1991:1).

This research heeds and affirms Lyotard's call for more localised, heterogeneous microanalysis situated in 'little narratives' (1984:60), as one constructive response to the criticism of the rejection of the grand narrative and the recoiling from totalising thought (Kellner, 1988:249). As will be discussed in the concluding chapter, this has particular importance in this work, where the research, far from being nihilist, actually documents one constructive example of the process of spiritual praxis and community action. Such a postmodern research framework, situated in epistemological understandings of discourse rather than the 'truth' of grand narratives (it will be argued) is important for exploring the illusive notion of spirituality: a notion marginalised by the modernist, scientific ways of knowing.

Ethical problematics

The concern with antifoundationalism and relativism centres not only on epistemological issues but also on ethical understandings.[29]

In our multicultural, ethically pluralistic society, where secularity and such religio-ethical-social value position such as Judaism, Christianity, Buddhism, and Islam need to co-exist, tolerance, respect for others and an acknowledgment of polycentrism replace previous notions of universal, absolute and exclusive worldviews (Charlesworth, 1993:165-6).[30]

In a liberal democratic society, the option is no longer consensus on a public or common morality, but rather a postmodern respect for 'difference', as Charlesworth explains,

> In essence, as has been said, the various groups may quite legitimately espouse and propagate their own specific religio-moral positions, but at the same time they cannot demand that they be imposed upon the whole community. They must agree to disagree (1993:167).

Whereas the project of modernity operated on a promise of absolutism, the postmodern world confronts bravely the concept of relativism. 'Assuming that the world is irreducibly pluralist, rendering the messages mutually communicable is its major problem' (Bauman, 1988:230). *That this is difficult is acknowledged.*

In bioethics, the question of reconciling incommensurable positions is translated into an ongoing search for a common ethical realm for 'moral strangers' which is able to incorporate the notion of 'difference'. The present postmodern bioethical challenge is not to inscribe closure through metaphysical or theological absolutism, but to explore the possibility of reconciling competing world views and values.

A beginning to such a dialogue can be seen by Engelhardt's (1991:11) notion of the prerequisite need for a 'will to morality' based on mutual respect and non-use of others without their consent, or Charlesworth's commitment to the liberal 'act of faith' in a society of autonomous, self-determining moral agents (1993:168), (notions developed further in chapter 13). The point is that this work recognises the problems of ethical relativism, not as insurmountable obstacles to postmodern theorising, but as a source of important ethico-epistemologico- political questions to be faced in a world where the foundational assumptions of the 'common content-full framework' (Engelhardt, 1991:xv) of religion, science and reason are under considerable suspicion.

Ruminating on reality

Postmodernism, like any other 'ism', is concerned with the two and a half thousand year old question: What is reality? As outlined previously, postmodernism is an ironic general social theory, which challenges the statements of grand theory which frame essentialist, metaphysical and epistemological, ontological assumptions, whilst at the same time seeking to make statements which provide provisional, local, insight into issues of power and 'difference'. Paradoxically, postmodernism wishes to explore 'reality' through language, whilst acknowledging the inescapable limits of language. A basic postmodern tenet, is that whilst reality may not be objectifiable, it is discussable, and not much more than this (Lemert, 1992:23).

As outlined in the introduction to this chapter, this discussability is of enormous importance, as postmodern notions of discourse have allowed the examination of a spiritual 'reality', which has not previously been easily accessible to research.

Such a position does not by inference necessitate as Bury (1986) suggests that postmodern analysis is unable to cope with the construction of a notion of reality. Rather, the postmodern approach applauds a plurality of realities. The point is, that any concept of objective reality, ultimately relates to fallible human frames of reference, and historically, culturally, and socially constructed epistemologies.[31]

One modernist concern (expressed as a criticism) which has been articulated about the postmodern approach to the construction of reality is that it suffers from a problem of incoherence, through logical contradiction and ideological ambiguity (Bury, 1986).[32] However, 'logical contradiction' and 'ideological ambiguity', although perceived as negative notions for modernists, are not necessarily interpreted with concern for postmodern writers. Indeed, it is at these very points of contradiction, ambiguity, and even paradox, that insight can be gained. Writers such as Huyssen (1990:268) would point to the 'contradictions' and 'contingencies', the 'tensions' and 'internal resistances' as the very ingredients in the modernist project which are worth exploring. This is not to deny as Boyne and Rattansi suggest that there is a great deal of coherence in postmodern thinking,

> There are important points of connection between the postmodernist decentring of the subject, its rejection of 'grand narratives', its espousal of 'local narratives', language games, and genealogies, its dread of totalising discourses leading to totalitarianism, and its political pluralism (1990:39).

The fear of nihilism

So far then, the generic criticisms of postmodernism, as they relate to this research have been examined and responded to. Finally, it is important to address criticisms in relation to the use of ideas developed by writers on deconstruction. As the 'will to power' behind this work is the desire to make a constructive contribution to the consideration of end-of-life bioethical issues, one modernist concern which is of particular interest is the often heard criticism that somehow deconstructive thinking will inevitably work to nihilist ends. Rather than indulge in argumentation on this issue, the actual doing of the research and the expression of the conclusions reached will, by way of example, stand as an indication that nihilism is not an inevitability.

Safeguards against the use of ideas associated with deconstruction being used only as an excuse for game-playing nihilism, are built into this work by the following three literary mechanisms. Firstly, as Norris clearly states, 'deconstruction affords no easy escape-route from the responsibility of authorship' (1989:189): my research text will stand as a text itself open to analysis and deconstruction. Indeed, Derrida who uses a process of deconstruction suggest that, rather than allowing the writer to escape into saying nothing, such a literary activity is actually 'the act of taking a position' (cited in Elam, 1994:90).[33]

Secondly, 'infinitized freeplay' is restricted by the obvious fact that the words of the texts exist, the words cannot be made to mean just anything (Norris, 1989:190).

Thirdly, intertextuality (the reading of one text through all the texts that the reader brings to it) (Worton and Still, 1990:1), will be developed through acknowledged academic discourses and research, appropriately related to this topic of analysis. The discourses which underpin my reading will be acknowledged and referenced.[34]

Conclusion

> The enlightenment is dead, Marxism is dead...and the author does not feel very well either (Smith cited in Lather, 1991:22).

As seen by the previous discussion, as exciting and attractive the ideas of postmodernism are for research, they are acknowledged to be at times problematic. This work takes up the challenge of exploring by doing, and seeks to contribute to the evolving body of work in this area. Inscribed in such a challenge, however, is a sense of both stimulation and trepidation, of enthusiasm and caution.

Mindful that 'in the text only the reader speaks' (Barthes cited in Lather, 1991:xx), this reading of postmodern problematics unapologetically seeks to inscribe a positive and useful openness to postmodern understandings. The response to the many criticisms is not to categorically reply that each point of concern has no substance. Within the many voices of the postmodern, there is the endless potential for nihilism, concealed metanarratives, confusion, and inaction. Based on the presupposition of a 'will to morality' and a 'will to contribute', this discussion privileges the possibility of using the insights gained with constructive intent. The humble hope is by actually getting in and doing postmodern research, some contribution can be made to the endless theorising on the inescapable problematics.

Far from being nihilistic, this work is situated in the paradoxes of seeking to construct through deconstructive thinking; offering a meaningful narrative in an absurdly meaningless world. This work is but one small offering to the altar of postmodernism, for as Becker explains,

> Who knows what form the forward momentum of life will take in the time ahead or what use it will make of our anguished searching. The most that any one of us can seem to do is to fashion something - an object or ourselves - and drop it into the confusion, make an offering of it, so to speak, to the life force (1973:285).

Notes

1 Lather (1991:105) explains this processs as the inscription of observable facts, recorded with transparent description, gathered through a clean separation of the interpreter and the interpreted.

2 According to Fox, knowledge, progress, truth and rationality constitute the unquestioned illusions of this epoch (Fox, 1991:722).

3 Although discussions of positivist ideas are now dated in the social sciences with recent literature on post-positivist development at the interface of theory, practice and research (Peile, 1994), this is not so with regard to the scientific epistemological foundations which underpin the bio-medical model (Cassell, 1991a; Fay, 1975; Lather, 1991; Ratcliff, 1989). Consequently, positivism, particularly as expressed in clinical medicine, will be taken as the dominant or 'first order' discourse with regard to illness and dying within our society.

4 Hart (1985:11) describes such an understanding as 'a dominant concern with the organic appearance of disease combined with a tendency to ignore, if not dismiss, the link between mind and body, between physical and mental well-being'. As will be seen later, not only is the emotional and mental link repressed but the whole notion of the spiritual dimension is at best marginalised, at worst deleted from such an understanding.

5 The scientific approach to death is referred to by Borges (1986:26) as the 'myth of salvation'. In describing the belief that science will conquer all, including death, Borges writes that, 'ironically enough, most people still cling to some semblance of the myth of salvation through science and even more specifically the illusion of medical salvation' (1986:26).

6 According to Smart (1993:91) 'the pursuit of order, promotion of calculability, fabrication and celebration of the "new", and faith in "progress" have been identified as pivotal features of modernity.' Turner

refers to the phenomenon of modernity as the 'great rational project of the 17th Century', and suggests that it is this very rationality which is now being challenged by postmodern writers as insufficiently coherent (Turner, 1990:16).

7 The postmodern concern with such metanarrtives as articulated in Lyotard's work, 'The Postmodern Condition' (1984) is summarised by Fraser and Nicholson (1988:376) when they write that, 'these "metanarratives" instantiate a specifically modern approach to the problem of legitimation. Each situates first-order discursive practices of inquiry and politics within a broader totalising metadiscourse which legitimates them...The story guarantees that some sciences and some politics have the right pragmatics and, so, are the right practices'. So legitimated, neither the Enlightenment Story or Science could be questioned as but one, fallible, construction of reality. Because of the perceived link between power and knowledge, Foucault sees any such totalising theory as dangerous, because of its power to dominate. The challenge according to Foucault is a 'hyper- and pessimistic' questioning of theory. On this issue he states that, 'not that everything is bad. If everything is dangerous, then we always have something to do. So my position leads not to apathy but to a hyper- and pessimistic activism' (Foucault in Rabinow, 1984:343). Lyotard acknowledges clearly the constructive contribution of the anti-totalising orientation of postmodern thought when he writes that, 'postmodern knowledge is not simply a tool of the authorities; it refines our sensitivity to differences and reinforces our ability to tolerate the incommensurable. Its principle is not the expert's homology, but the inventor's paralogy' (1984:xxv).

8 Philosophers from the Frankfurt School were leaders in the critique of the Age of Reason which included a critique of the scientific method. Values of domination and control, rather than neutrality are seen to underpin the epoch (Borges, 1986:27). In place of one unifying progressive teleology, postmodern writers such as Featherstone point to the evidence of 'complex incommensurable teleologies, of heterogeneity in social, society and aesthetic experience' (1988:209). Indeed the very notion of rationality itself was rejected. Brubaker's work, based on a Weberian critique of the 'iron cage' of capitalism, points to the disjunction between formal and substantial rationality, and argues that to the extent that ends and beliefs diverge, so too will judgments of rationality and irrationality. There are, he concludes, inherent limits to the rationality of individual action and the rationality of the social order (Brubaker, 1984).Marcuse (1972), similarly points out the irrationality of modern western rationality, by making clear the totalitarian nature of such technologically controlled, supposedly democratic, 'Reason'. According to Marcuse, 'the web of domination has become the web of Reason itself, and this society is fatally entangled in it' (Marcuse, 1972:138). Horkheimer, a writer from the German Frankfurt School, similarly debunks the whole notion of rationality in an essay titled, 'The End of Reason' (1978). For Horkheimer, a neutral objective rationality cannot be extracted from its intricate link with the historical,

political and sociological influences of society. He states that, 'to be sure, reason cannot hope to keep aloof from history and to intuit the true order of things, as ontological ideologies contend...ideology consists more in what men (sic), are like than in what they believe - in their mental constrictedness, their complete dependence upon associations' (1978:47).

9 Indeed postmodern theorising is seen as a response to the shattering of such myths of modernity (Smart, 1993). The promise of modernity did not come to realisation, as Smart (1993:91) explains, 'modernity, in turn, has become the focus of increasing critical reflection in the course of the twentieth century. The benefits and securities assumed to be a corollary of the development of modernity have become matters of doubt, the possibility of their realisation, if not their desirability, the subject of question and criticism as faith in the doctrine of progress has been dissipated'.

10 Jameson (1984:xix) in the forward to Lyotard's book *The Postmodern Condition*, describes such a vision of science and technology as 'a search, not for consensus, but very precisely for 'instabilities', a practice of paralogism, in which the point is not to reach agreement but to undermine from within the very framework in which the previous 'normal science' had been conducted.'

11 Lather (1991:vii) speaks of reality as 'a text, subject to multiple interpretations, multiple readings, multiple uses', signifying not only the different socio-historico-cultural influences on theorists but also their particular 'will to power'.

12 Perhaps this is because definitions are problematic in postmodern thinking, as Elam explains, (1994:4), they 'threaten to function like final answers which erase the fact that there were ever any questions asked in the first place; their status becomes unshakeable, almost natural, and rarely if ever interrogated. Thus..it would be a mistake to offer up easy definitions.'

13 Best and Kellner (1991:58) sum up this relationship between discourse and power when they articulate the Foucaluldian position that 'in any society, discourse is power because the rules determining discourse enforce norms of what is rational, sane, or true, and to speak form outside these rules is to risk marginalisation and exclusion'.

14 Such medical control, as Borges points out (1986:28) is disguised both under the rubric of caring and protection and as an ideology of excellence based on a desire to serve and protect.

15 Authors such as Zola (1975) would see the power behind the biomedical discourse invading all areas of living as well as dying, through a process known as the 'medicalization' of life. Zola suggests that this process operates 'by making medicine and the labels "health" and "illness" relevant to an ever increasing part of human existence' (1975:83). As the dying trajectory by its very nature implies health problems it is particularly vulnerable to such 'medicalizing' influences.

16 According to Derrida, deconstruction is neither an analysis nor a critique, nor a method, or an act or even an operation (Elam, 1994:12). His description is even more elusive, as seen by his statement that

'deconstruction takes place, it is an event that does not await the deliberation, consciousness, or organisation of a subject, or even of modernity' (cited in Elam, 1994:12).

17 The 'known' in this case refers to the more established methodologies of the social sciences. Such research would have, at least, have had its modus operandi legitimated, by an interpretative community comfortable with such a research orientation. For as Foucault argues, any contribution to 'the techniques and procedures accorded value in the acquisition of truth', are not absolute, but rather the result of the 'effects of power' on truth production, directly a function of 'the status of those who are charged with saying what counts as true' (cited in Rabinow, 1984:73). Such 'effects of power' in the present discussion, are in relation to the process of academic legitimation, (or otherwise), of frameworks of research, and in the case of this work, postmodern explorations of knowledge.

18 As stated by Engelhardt and Wildes (1994:141) 'The post-modern context is defined by the realisation that this difficulty is insuperable. A particular, canonical, contextfull, philosophical account of morality cannot be identified.'

19 Such critics describe the postmodern approach as an 'ephemeral fashion', just the invention of paid university theorists to further their careers (Pawley, 1986), or more scathingly as the 'malaise at the heart of contemporary culture' (Featherstone, 1988:195).

20 Whether viewed as the nascent state of modernity which searches for new presentations of the unpresentable, (Lyotard, 1984:79-81), the cultural logic of late capitalism (Jameson, 1991), or an embryonic episteme which seeks to inscribe heterogeneity, inconclusiveness, and complexity (Elam, 1994), theories of the postmodern can be used 'with astonishing frequency in a surprising variety of ways' (Gare, 1995:4).

21 Authors such as Gare (1995:33) fear that such a demise of the master discourse on truth actually leads to the disempowerment of people and a breakdown of 'genuine' praxis. Such ideas will be countered in the final chapter on bioethical reflections. Douglas (1986) argues that it is this very inability to contribute to the solution of problems, that leads intellectuals to an inward journey of relativism and by implication, nihilism.

22 Rawlinson (1987:374) summarises this Foucaultian critique of totalising knowledge clearly when she states that such an approach 'calls into question classical notions of the universality of truth by establishing the historicity of all knowledge; it undermines any pose of scientific neutrality or disinterestedness by exposing the ineluctable intertwining of systems for the production of knowledge with systems for the deployment of power and force; and it educes a reexamination of what is happening when actual human subject are formed by institutionalised procedures of education, testing, certification, evaluation, regulation, and treatment.'

23 As Pierce (1991:70) states on this point, 'before we become overly pessimistic regarding the possibility of ethics or political theory, it must be noticed that the postmodern disparagement of universalistic claims applies only to discussions that try to capture truths about the world.'

24 Mumby (1988:137) suggests that 'theory building should not be conceived as the search for essences, but as a way of contributing to the continual flow of interesting and useful things that can be said about the world.'

25 Many postmodern authors see the problem as being one of writers being overwhelmed by the difficulties of the intellectual task of operating in such a crisis of meaning (Kellner, 1988:266); Elam, 1994:7), and so either oppose postmodernism outright (Bury, 1986), or seek such oxymoronic solutions, as an alternative postmodern grand theory (Gare, 1995; Boyne and Rattansi, 1990:40). There are representatives from all sides of the political spectrum from 'neo-conservative' to 'progressive', who reject the postmodern questioning of the grand narrative (Lather, 1991:114). Difference is alive and well, it is obvious, even among those who fear relativism, and adhere to foundationalism and a belief in grand theory. Difference, and relativism, are actualities, both for those who oppose and espouse the anti-foundational, postmodern ethos.

26 Which as Elam explains, 'allows us to imagine other political spaces - spaces of political otherness. This is an acknowledgment that politics is not an order of meaning, that politics will not come to an end and explain what other people are, what their otherness means...There are differences, they arise, always more of them...This is a depressing thought for people who don't like politics, who don't like difference, who just want to get it over with and make everyone happy.' (1994:85).

27 Indeed, it is acknowledged that the postmodern ethos with its emphasis on uncertainty, and complexity, must be uncomfortable to those who seek the ideological, authoritative, totalitarian crutch of knowingness, and of absolute truth. Such discomfort can be expressed both as an excuse for paralysing nihilism, and/or a call to understanding based on deconstructive difference, outside the form of modernist reasoning of what Lather would refer to as the binary logics of certainty, non-contradiction, totality and linearity (1991:xvi).

28 There is even the suspicion that postmodern writers may cloak the very contradiction of inscribing truth while critiquing foundationalism. Indeed, Rorty charges Foucault with an ambiguous epistemology which is 'loaded to the brim with truth claims' (Barrett, 1991:145).

29 Ethical judgments, for example, can no longer be believed to be absolutely and categorically true, as in the preceding, deontological tradition of such moral theorists as Kant (Johnstone, 1994:54), or in the absolutist orientation of such philosophers as Descartes, Spinoza, Hegel, Schopenhauer (McCarl Nielsen, 1990:3). Moral 'truth', is no longer seen as an absolute notion which can be arrived at by the detached, liberated, mental wanderings of the individual philosopher.

30 As Engelhardt explains, (1991:xiv), 'the postmodern age is the age of moral strangers', characterised by a lack of a central concrete moral vision, replaced by disparate moralities.

31 In short, as Nicolson and McLaughlin (1987:112) explain, 'while natural knowledge is about nature, the assessment of natural knowledge is a social process'. Charlesworth expresses this idea clearly when he writes, 'the idea

that there are pure 'data' is likewise incoherent. What we call the "facts" or the "data" are a product of the meeting between a framework of ideas, expectations, principles of interpretation on one hand, and the observable world on the other hand, so that what the scientist observes is a 'construction' - something that is made up out of elements from our side;so to speak, and elements from the side of the external world' (1989:9).

32 Indeed, a great deal of the postmodern writing is obscure in meaning, and difficult to interpret, perhaps because it is written with the intent to disrupt. It is important, nevertheless, not to throw the baby of understanding out with the bathwater of verbosity.

33 Any reading is always provisionally open to further deconstruction of its own operative concepts (Norris, 1982:48). My interpretations will be open to review by what Fish refers to as 'the interpretive community' (Arac, 1990:47). However, interpretations in this view are never intrinsically valid or invalid: assumptions and beliefs will be quickly assented to, accepted, and ratified by those in the community who hold the same assumptions.

34 Mumby (1988:115) reinforces this point when he writes, 'interpreting a text is not an entirely pluralistic enterprise in which every interpretation, however idiosyncratic or superficial, is considered to be equally worthy of consideration.'

3 Engaging in the research

This chapter examines the pragmatic and practical aspects of conducting this study within the context of the theoretical discussion of the postmodern approach. The intent of this discussion is to move from a theoretical abstract discussion of postmodern notions, to a consideration of the local, contextual, restricted theorising of postmodern social inquiry.

Recap and summary

To recapitulate on the discussion so far, this research will be situated in a postmodern approach with particular emphasis placed on the notions associated with discourse and deconstruction.

This leads to a desire to play with ideas, explore the related literature, draw connections between the focus questions and recent research, understand notions of discourse, power and subjectivity, develop questions, and seek innovative frameworks for reflection on these issues. I am not proposing a strict, tightly defined methodology, but rather one which uses the insights of writers on deconstruction to generate ideas about my topic.

From the purely theoretical to the particular

According to Fairclough (1989:13; 1992:56), a major limitation of the work on power and discourse, by such writers as Foucault, is the purely theoretical nature of its contribution. The suggestion is that such understandings need to be 'operationalised in the analysis of particular instances of discourse' (ibid). This research takes up such a challenge by consideration of the postmodern theoretical understanding of power and discourse in relation to the discursive practices of a particular community based hospice organisation, Karuna

Hospice Service (KHS).

The hospice phenomenon is only a few decades old, so understandably the research in this relatively new field is scarce (Petrosino, 1988:29). Within the limited research that has been completed, there is scant research focusing on community volunteer programs such as KHS (Siebold, 1992:158). Many researchers have been concerned about this lack of research in the hospice area (Dush, 1988b; Lamers, 1988; Mount, 1985; Paradis, 1988). Predominantly, the hospice literature is descriptive, with a strong orientation to medically based discourses (Siebold, 1992:158).

Consequently, there are calls within the literature for researchers to marry theoretical assumptions with applied research (Lamers, 1988:5; Paradis, 1988:69). This work is a response to such a call for research.

Meeting the criteria of postmodern social inquiry

In keeping with the postmodern tenets outlined in previous chapters, notions associated with writers who use deconstruction and insights from within the literature on discourse will be applied in an attempt to distil provisional, local, contextual insights of questions relating to ideas of the 'uniqueness' and 'resistance' of KHS.

This research, meets the criteria of postmodern social inquiry, as outlined by Seidman and Wagner (1992:7). Firstly, it is explicitly practical. The focus is on the discourse of practice, of intervention, of service provision by a community based palliative care service, known as the Karuna Hospice Service. It is anticipated that the insights developed may have practical implications for understanding death and dying within our society. It is 'practical research in situated location(s)' which will hopefully yield contextual insights, not 'categories of "universal" truths' (Aronowitz, 1992:314).

Secondly, this social inquiry has moral intent. The expectation is that such research will make a contribution to bioethical epistemology, the palliative care movement, and the normative enterprise of exploring the possibility of 'death with dignity' (Kubler-Ross, 1969; 1974; 1975; Morison, 1975a; 1975b; Poss, 1981; Ramsey, 1975; Saunders, 1993).

Thirdly, such research is contextual and restricted in focus, incorporating local, rather than general, stories. This work does not aspire to contribute to a grand theory of the care of the dying, but rather to analyse and to reflect upon a particular discourse at one point in time. Such a study 'would be respectful of the complex experiences of the people under study' (Seidman, 1992:71): a local narrative concerned with articulating the viewpoint and concern of those involved in Karuna Hospice Service at one particular point in their history.

Fourthly, this research will be concerned with the notions people convey in talking about their situation. The data collection has been carried out through open-ended, non-structured interviews with a cross-section of participants from this organisation. It is, quite simply, 'what people, in concrete settings, learn to say and do say, about their condition' (Lemert, 1992:41).

Studies of discourse are not uncommon in the field of health and medicine research, as seen by the following examples. Clark and Mishler (1992:344-372), focusing on studies of medical discourse, conversational storytelling, and narrative, analysed the exercise of authority in clinical encounters. Fisher and Todd's work (1986a; 1986b) relates studies of discourse to institutional contexts, in particular, they are interested in how the institution of medicine lends power to physicians to control the interaction with their patients. Taped conversations between patient and doctor were the text for examining discourse in the work of Fisher (1991:157-182). Waitzkin (1989:220-238) used a critical theory of medical discourse to examine ideology and social control in the social context of medical encounters.

An example of a similar model is seen in the work of Mumby and Stohl (1991:313-332).[1] They used deconstructive analysis in order to understand how discourse reproduces meaning structures organisationally.

Within the bioethical literature, such a postmodern use of discourse in research would be considered both innovative and perhaps a challenge to mainstream empirical methodology, and the priority given to philosophical reflection based on principlism. There is, however, some evidence of a beginning of a new direction in bioethical research which shares with this research not only the inclusion of Eastern theological /spiritual perspectives, but also the importance and usefulness of the notion of discourse for research. This change in direction can be seen by such examples as Clooney's (1995) writing on the moral discourse of a Hindu community, Ratanakul's (1986; 1988) and Florida's (1994) exploration of the contribution of Buddhist thought to bioethics, and Newell's (1991; 1992; 1995) examination of the bioethical issues associated with disability through an understanding of discourse.

The discussion so far has been broadly theoretical, providing the focus (Chapter 1), frameworks (Chapter 2), and overview for this study, with examples of similar research (present chapter), so as to situate this study firmly in postmodern epistemological understandings. The task of the rest of this chapter is to describe in detail the practical operationalisation of this study. This discussion will cover the 'doing of the research'; exploring such issues as defining the texts for research, gaining ethical clearance, establishing preliminary and ongoing relationships with KHS, and collecting, shaping and giving meaning to the data.

Defining the texts

With such a process in mind, a number of texts, both written and spoken, were gathered. This parallels Fairclough's working definition of text, when he refers to,

> ...the term text ... for both written texts and 'spoken texts'; a spoken text is simply what is said in a piece of spoken discourse, but I shall generally use the term for a written transcription of what is said (Fairclough, 1989:24).

For the purpose of this work, the texts, so defined, include,

1 The Karuna Hospice Service Vision and Values Statement.

2 Detailed verbatim scripts of interviews with organisational members and clients of Karuna Hospice Service and outside health professionals who have had an association, either past or present, with this service.

Whilst the KHS Vision and Values Statement is an easily accessible, short, two page document, the gathering of interview material is a more complex process and hence will now be examined more fully.

Exact replication of such spoken texts were made through audio recordings. The process of developing the 'spoken texts' was through open-ended, non-directive interviewing with individuals who have had a significant association with KHS.

The aim of such text creation was a postmodern interest to explore difference and discourse, not a modernist concern to collect objective data. As Mulkay advocates (1985:8-11), the challenge in developing such postmodern research texts is to be open to interpretive complexity, mindful of the possibility of engaging in multiple, non-linear, polyvocal, and multi-levelled readings. Consequently, the aim of selecting participants was to achieve heterogeneity of discursive expression. As comprehensive a sample as possible was selected from within the population available. For this reason, a full range of individuals from both within and outside this service was included; those presently employed and those with a past working history with KHS; those who had had positive experiences and those carrying emotional pain from their association with this organisation; professionals and non-professionals; volunteers, clients, administrators, nurses, a doctor, and a spiritual leader. This insured that as many different perspectives as possible were integrated into the language/texts.

In particularly, I was impressed by the integrity of key players who suggested (without prompting) the names of individuals who had been marginalised and who consequently felt a degree of emotional pain about the service. Such interviews added a richness and depth to the research data.

The number of interviewees was limited to fifteen (15), although one was not taken verbatim because of recorder problems. These interviewees can be divided into the following categories -

1 The Director of KHS.

2 Four (4) Nurses -
One (1) originally a key player in the organisation's development but no longer employed by KHS.
Two (2) employed at that time by KHS.
One (1) an oncology nurse employed at a major hospital who represented the only person the researcher could find who expressed critical views of this organisation.

3 Two (2) Administrative Staff -
One (1) a key player in introducing administrative procedures to the

organisation but no longer employed by KHS. One (1) the administrator of KHS at the time of the interview.

4 One (1) Palliative Care Medical Practitioner who had a long term involvement with KHS.

5 One (1) Volunteers Co-ordinator, a significant player in the formation of this service.

6 Two (2) members of the KHS board of management.
One (1) a solicitor and one (1) a psychologist, both long term members of this organisation.

7 One (1) community development worker who was no longer associated with KHS but who had participated in this organisation's early development.

8 One (1) volunteer who had a long term association with this service and who is presently an active participant.

9 Two (2) clients, each with a family representative.
(Counted here as two (2) interviews.)

Perhaps due to the intimate nature of the interviewing situation, these interviews lasted from one to one and a half hours and produced an enormous amount of text.

As outlined previously, these fifteen interviews incorporated a great deal of heterogeniety, with a multiplicity of voices expressing a complexity of view-points. In short, there was a richness of material emerging which was useful for later interpretation. Although fifteen (15) interviews may appear a small number in comparison to some quantitative research, the length, depth and richness of these interviews provided more than adequate data for this research with its focus on discourse. Blum (1970:84) describes this as the research practice of developing data through intense interaction with a small group of participants rather than using extensive sampling method.

Each interview when transcribed, it is important to note, varied from six (6) to ten (10) thousand words, producing an immense amount of data. As stated by McCracken (1988:17) the rationale behind using interviews for research is the principle that 'less is more'. That is, 'it is more important to work longer, and with greater care, with a few people than more superficially with many of them' (McCracken, 1988:17).[2]

Other studies using complete transcripts of interviews as a bases for analysis have used as few as two interviews. Such an example is seen in the case of Fisher and Todd (1986a:29), who examined the medicalization of social problems in physician interaction with patients. In the research literature there appears to be enormous variation in the number of participants used in studies relying on recorded interviews. There was, however, ample evidence of work which ranged from the just cited case of two to about twenty participants, as seen by the examples documented in the notes to this chapter. [3]

It is also important to note that although there were only two (2) interviews undertaken with the families who were cared for by KHS, the positive nature of the information which emerged has been affirmed many times over by the 'stories' told to me in informal discussions by many other families cared for by this service. It has been my experience that those cared for by KHS are always enthusiastic to share their 'stories' and do so with a sense of high regard and gratitude for the organisation. Such 'stories' have emerged from the most unlikely places, for example, from a member of the ethics review board to which this research was submitted for approval and a receptionist at the local musical instrument shop.

The terminally ill or dying have been described in the literature on research methods as a vulnerable population, with discussion centring on whether such groups should or should not be asked to participate in research[4] (Raudonis, 1992). With the difficulty of these ethical questions in mind, it was decided that the inclusion of this small number of clients would suffice, as their interviews would be situated in the knowledge of the many other consistent and ongoing positive client stories which have arisen from the other sources just described.[5]

The interviewing process

Most of the interviews were conducted in coffee shops, or in the work place of the participants. Clients of KHS were interviewed in their own home. Such home interviews added to the very enriching experience for the researcher by contextualising the spoken text to the situation of the dying person. Friends calling to visit, children moving in and out of the room of the patient, a cat on the end of the bed, the lack of medical paraphernalia, and the many personal possessions that spoke of the patient's individuality, were all important paralinguistic clues that affirmed the comments made about the process of dying in one's own home.

Interviewees were enthusiastic to participate,[6] and many spent considerable time before the interviews thinking through issues to discuss and writing down points to raise. All of the interviews were taped on a small hand-held tape recorder. Although the presence of the recorder was felt initially by both the participant and the interviewer, this seemed to dissipate quickly. So minimal was the presence of the tape recorder that often the 'click' at the end of a tape came as a surprise, awakening the participant to its presence.

For one interview, the tape did not work and the recording was lost. To compensate, I wrote down all that could be recalled from the interview after the session ended. This material, taken from an interview in a patient's home, has been treated as back-up information, rather than as a verbatim account.[7]

The research focus was explained to all the participants. Preceding each interview, the participant was provided with a statement outlining such a focus in written form. The starting point for each interview was an invitation to the interviewee to explore whether they did or did not believe KHS was different from other hospice services in Brisbane and why. The interviewee was encouraged to use actual examples of experiences both at KHS and also at other organisations, which would convey some idea to the researcher of the uniqueness or otherwise of this service and its relationship to other organisations. This discussion usually followed a short introduction where the participant situated themselves occupationally and historically within the context of KHS.

This short introduction served not only to 'set the stage'; so to speak, but also to relax any of the interviewees' angst and to start the flow of conversation.

A non-directive approach was taken to interviewing in an attempt to capture as spontaneously as possible a diverse and open sample of the various discourses operating in and around KHS.[8] The agenda and direction of the discussion were considered as important an expression of the participants discourse as their response to the questions asked. As will be seen in the later section on research findings, the topics the participants chose to place on the agenda for discussion during these interviews came to direct the analysis as much as any question asked by the interviewer.

Exploring the social relations of the research act

So far in this discussion, the focus has been on the 'gazed upon'. The concern has been with giving a description of the participants and outlining why they were chosen.

This is, however, only one part of the research picture, if viewed through a postmodern lens. Postmodern social inquiry has an understanding of the social construction of knowledge that suggests that the social context of the 'gazer' is as important as that of the 'gazed upon'. As has been outlined in previous discussions (Chapter 2), the postmodern approach challenges the whole notion of the neutrality of the scientific method. The notion that the researcher can somehow stand outside the research process and gaze objectively at the participants is rejected. In its place is an *episteme* which accepts that no knowledge can be obtained or interpreted outside the meaning made possible by the research act. The values, skills and meaning making the researcher brings to the data collection is seen to be as vital an influence on the outcome as any characteristics of the participants. In a cycle of mutual influence, the researcher and participants are seen to impact on each others thoughts and agendas.

This cycle of mutual influence quite dramatically touched not only the dynamics of data collection but actually altered the very questions being asked by this research. As will be demonstrated in the following discussion, the participants' thoughtful comments not only directed and enriched the research material, but also led to a different interpretation of the original research focus. Far from any positivist notion of the clean separation of researcher and participant, this example of postmodern research acknowledges and prizes the mutual engagement of both researcher and participants in the production of ideas which emerged from this study. This mutual engagement will now be explored from three important perspectives: firstly, the influence of the researcher; secondly, a description of the factors impacting on data collection during the interviews; and thirdly, the impact of the participants on the research questions. Connecting all these perspectives is the notion of the social relations of the research act (Lather, 1991:91), which signifies the active participation of both the interviewer and interviewees in the production of knowledge.

Mutual engagement - the influence of the researcher

As it would be an impossible task to truly enumerate the multitudinous influences any researcher would bring to their work, it will have to suffice to situate myself as a bioethicist with a background in social work who brings an interest in ideas of palliative care, the philosophy of science, psychology, sociology and spirituality.

Perhaps a more convincing insight into the assumptions underpinning this work can be seen by the actual interpretation of the data and the theoretical synthesis of insights so gained: in short, the actual writing up of the work.

It is important to point out that two firmly held value positions underpin this work: firstly, the ethic of care, and secondly, a concern about the impact of the 'technological imperative' (Fuchs, 1968) on the dying experience.

The central notion of the ethic of care is a philosophical commitment to a discourse which universalises the emotion of caring (Noddings, 1984). There is, to use a Foucaultian styled phrase, a 'will to care'. Such an ethic incorporates three dimensions as central to developing understanding, these being, firstly, an emphasis on individual uniqueness, secondly, the acceptance of the appropriateness of emotions in dialogue, and thirdly, the cultivation of the capacity for empathy (Fonow and Cook, 1991:10). Although abstract rules and principles are acknowledged to have a place in ethical reasoning, these are not seen as the supreme or only means to moral judgment. Of equal importance is a compassionate understanding of the individual's life space, as only the emotions of empathy and caring can provide.

The importance of context and the central value of the emotion of caring will thus be implicit assumptions underpinning this work. This perspective is reinforced by my background as a social worker and my work as a palliative care educator.

Later discussion in Chapter 8 will elaborate in detail my concern about the impact of the 'technological imperative' (Fuch, 1968:192) on the dying experience.

So far, the influence of the researcher has been discussed in very general terms. This influence will now be contextualised to the process of interviewing which has been flagged as the second topic of focus when considering the dynamic of the mutual engagement of both researcher and participants in the production of ideas.

Mutual engagement - the dynamics of the interviews

The postmodern approach incorporates a respect for self-reflexivity and hence acknowledges the influence, both verbal and non-verbal, of the researcher, both in the production and the interpretation of the texts. The notion is that there can be no linear distinction between the interviewing process and data analysis.

Of particular importance to this interviewing process was the researcher's respect and enthusiasm for the work of KHS.[9] Both intellectually and emotionally, the researcher brought to these interviews a sense of high regard for those being interviewed, as well as a very positive appreciation of the achievements of the service. In most of the areas under discussion, there was a sharing of values between the interviewer and interviewee.[10] Interestingly, such a positive orientation, rather than privileging only the 'good stories', facilitated a richer, more complex understanding of issues, often including, the expression of quite painful and sensitive emotions and insights. One interviewee confided, when sharing such information, that she would only do so knowing that the researcher would treat with respect the information offered. It appeared that my commitment to KHS provided a foundation of trust, which allowed for the expression of quite difficult issues.

With the exception of the two broad areas of focus (uniqueness and resistance), I came to the interviews with the 'will to listen and reflect'.[11] These interviews reflect basic counselling skills of active listening[12] and reflection[13] (Tomm, 1988).

The interviews came to a sense of closure when both interviewee and researcher felt the topic had been exhausted. Many of the participants commented on how much they enjoyed the experience of taking part. Some of the participants commented that the interviews allowed them to discuss, in a cathartic fashion, pain they had been carrying for a considerable time about the service. At times, participants cried during the interview, (the tape was turned off at such times), when dealing with sensitive topics. However, these participants expressed an appreciation for being able to explore such sensitive issues. The research process was seen by the participants to be both positive and, at times, healing. Participants expressed the notion that these interviews gave them a feeling of being listened to, and this was most appreciated.

Participants were invariably articulate and reflective, bringing to the interviews many years of ruminating over the topics under consideration. At times there were discussions which individuals did not want to be recorded. The tape recorder was turned off during these discussions, and the material was not included in the language/texts. The right of the interviewee to withdraw any or all of their statements was stressed throughout this research process, however, there was no request to edit information.

The data, it has been shown, was collected through the medium of the mutual engagement in interviews of a researcher who was respectful and enthusiastially supportive of KHS and the many participants who were equally as enthusiastic to share their thoughts about this service. Interviewing skills, articulate and intelligent interviewees, the intimacy of a long interview, the flexibility of a non-directive approach, and mutual respect and trust between interviewer and interviewee were some of the ingredients which impacted on this research process.

Such a mutual engagement, as has been previously suggested, was not restricted just to the collection of data. Indeed, as will now be discussed, participants' comments were far more influential than simply providing the material for analysis. They were also instrumental in interpreting the very notions upon which the research focused.

Mutual engagement - the research focus

Part of the original research focus was 'What is the uniqueness of KHS?' When this question was asked of one participant, his response was,

> When you set it up as being unique it becomes elitist, and I don't see Karuna as being elite. I just see it as being a group of ordinary committed people who are trying to offer a compassionate service and compassion is something universal and it is practised all over the world.

This participants' criticism of my use of the term 'unique' was accepted for the documentation of this study. The word 'difference' was substituted, and valued as useful and important by all those interviewed, both inside and outside this service organisation. In comparison to the distinction made in positivistic research between the researcher and participants (Lather, 1991:105), this postmodern research acknowledges the mutual engagement of both researcher and participants in the production of ideas. The influence of the researcher, the dynamics of the interview, and the impact of the participant on the reseach agenda were all shown to be factors central to understanding this process of mutual engagement.

Stage 1 analysis

Once the interviews were completed, the next step was to transcribe and analyse the interviews.The taped interviews were transcribed verbatim, making individual language/texts approximately twenty to twenty-five (20-25) pages long. These notes were referenced with initials of the speakers and page and line numbers. There were one hundred and twenty-four pages of completed language/text.

Stage one of the analysis of these texts, was a thematic analysis of significant statements. As this research was concerned with discursive practices, such an analysis used the exact words of the participants, not abstract concepts developed from such transcripts. All ideas expressed were included, with one interview at a time being used to create categories and with subsequent interviews analysed in such a way as to build on these or to create new categories. This was a challenging process for, as Whyte (1982:120-1) explains, such interviews produce a voluminous amount of data which, unlike structured questionnaires, 'do not automatically order' with the real possibility that 'as the numbers of interviews pile up (the researcher)...may find himself (herself) swamped.'

Such a process of thematic analysis of these language/texts was obviously restricted to, and guided by, the exact words of the interviewees. The research material, to a degree, determined what could eventually be said about the issues under focus. However, this is only part of the story. Because this research was postmodern in orientation, such an organisation of the material gathered was seen as an early 'reading' of the research findings. As Worton and Still suggest, 'what is produced at the moment of reading is due to the cross-fertilisation of the packaged textual material ... by all the texts which the reader brings to it' (Worton and Still, 1990:1).

Stage 2 analysis

This material was then collapsed into thirty-five (35) pages of compact statements. The reason for this process was to identify patterns of repetition in the material, and similar statements were eliminated but the reference recorded.

Key words were highlighted to draw out themes and provide an overview. Categories were reviewed in terms of the goals of the research with, at times, new categories being created.

Some of the material was diagrammatically represented for clarity. An outline of the significant ideas emerging from this process was sketched with a set of discussion points isolated for further development.

The second stage of the process was important in playing with, and exploring the potential of, the material for research insights. It provided a structure and an analytical process for the research, but script from the first stage was ultimately found to be more useful for citing and recording sections of the language/texts. While the elimination of repetition helped to develop a good overview, it simultaneously removed the subtlety of meaning of many of the statements. The examples provided in the discussion of the research findings were taken from the first stage of the analysis.

Presenting the research

Before concluding this chapter, it is important to set the stage for the following presentation of the research findings by explaining the format such a presentation will take. The exact quotes of interviewees will be used for reference through the following discussions. For reasons of confidentiality, participants have been assured that no identifying information will accompany such quotes. These quotations will not be referenced individually as the full appendices (because of reasons of privacy and confidentiality) cannot be made available for publication. The abbreviation (EQ) will be used to identify all exact quotes in the text. Such a format which includes direct quotes from participants has been used in publishing the results of other research projects in the area of hospice and palliative care. Munley's book (1983) *The Hospice Alternative*, and McNulty and Holderby's book, *Hospice: A Caring Challenge* (1983), are two such examples.

Conclusion

This chapter, has explored the many influences on how the data for this research was shaped and given meaning, with the researcher's voice being seen as but 'one among others creating meaning' (Gitlin cited in Lather, 1991:91). This material forms the basis of the more complete description/ interpretation which unfolds in the following discussions.

Such a story will inescapably inscribe as much about the researcher as it does about the organisation it seeks to understand. In accepting responsibility for such authorship, it is my humble wish that I do justice to the sensitive and insightful understandings the participants have brought to this study.

Notes

1 This is seminal work in this area, however, as Mumby (1988:99) states, 'To date, only a handful of organisational theorists have even begun to study the relationship among language, ideology, and power in organisations'.

2 McCraken (1988:17) in fact suggest that 'for many research projects eight (8) respondents will be perfectly sufficient'.

3 In an exploration of the caring behaviours of hospice nurses, Hull (1991:63) interviewed ten (10) families. Ten (10) audio taped interviews were also completed for the research of Raudonis (1995:59) in a study which explored the development of empathic nurse-patient relationships between terminally ill adult hospice nurses and their hospice patients. In earlier hospice research (used as the basis of a doctoral dissertation), Raudonis (1991) studied such empathy from the patients perspective using interviews with fourteen (14) patients in their homes. In quite recent and similar Ph D research, Ross (1994:445) explored the topic of spirituality by using taped interviews with twelve (12) nurses. Hyman and Bulkin (1990:39) chose to interview seventeen (17) practising physicians when examining the incentives and disincentives for referring patients to hospice. Britten's work (1991:83) used tape recordings of twenty (20) interviews with medical consultants when exploring physicians' views about patient access to general practice records. Degner and associates (1991:246) developed a list of critical nursing behaviours in the care of the dying through interviews recorded verbatim with ten (10) nurse educators and ten (10) experienced palliative care nurses.

4 Kane (1986:6) elaborates on this issue when he states that 'from an ethical standpoint, one is concerned about being overly voyeuristic and intrusive.

From a practical standpoint any of the subjects may quickly reach a stage where they can no longer tolerate the burden of a lengthy questionnaire, if they respond at all.' According to Wilkinson (1986:75) terminally ill patients may be 'unable or unwilling to use precious time and energy to answer researchers' questions.'

5 Before commencing the interviewing process, ethical clearance was obtained from the Behavioural and Social Sciences Ethical Review Committee of the University of Queensland. Voluntary participation, sensitive interviewing, adequate information about the research, the right of withdrawal at any stage, confidentiality, and access to relevant data obtained were all considered issues of moral relevance for this research. The vulnerable group which was of concern included the 'subjects in a dependent relationship with the investigator' who may have felt some obligation to participate (BSSERC, 1993:8). Such a group included the patients of the hospice service. In an attempt to remove or minimise coercion, such participants were informed of the research, and an offer extended to include their valuable experience. However, the initiative was left to the patient to approach a member of the hospice service team or myself if they considered the participation in the research appropriate. Each participant in the research was given a written summary sheet on the objectives of the study and a written consent form. All participants, engaged in a detailed discussion on ethical issues to be considered before their involvement, read the written summary and signed the consent form before participation.

6 The notion of meaning making and spirituality surfaced throughout these interviews. Research by Fife (1994:316) indicates that, similarly to this work, 'meaning is a concept that persons seem willing to discuss freely.'

7 Such notes, although not seen as satisfactory as recordings, are accepted as a legitimate mechanism for recording interviews and are chosen as a preferred method by some researchers (Whyte, 1982:118).

8 Burgess (1982:107) provides a description of the aims of an unstructured interview which echoes the direction of this work and that includes, 'the opportunity for the researcher to probe deeply, to uncover new clues, to open up new dimensions of a problem and to secure vivid, accurate, inclusive accounts from informants that are based on personal experience.'

9 My previous positive relationship with this organisation overcame the problem which first confronts researchers looking at any service and this is the task of establishing a working relationship based on a sense of familiarity (Blum, 1970:83).

10 Throughout the literature on data collection by interviewing such familiarity is seen as a positive factor (Burgess, 1982:108; Phillips, 1971:129).

11 Burgess (1982:107) records that 'interviewers need to be good listeners as well as questioners.'

12 Active listening is very different from just hearing what the other person has to say. Bolton (1987:32) explains this difference when he writes, 'Listening, then, is the combination of hearing what the other person says

and a suspenseful waiting, an intense psychological involvement with the other.'

13 Bolton (1987:50) links the art of active listening with the capacity to respond reflectively when he states, 'The art of good listening involves the ability to respond reflectively. In a reflective response, the listener restates the feeling and/or content of what the speaker has communicated and does so in a way that demonstrates understanding and acceptance.'

4 Setting the stage by stating the difference

Having established the epistemological assumptions underpinning this research, this chapter will now begin to explore the 'talk' arising from the first research question.

Translating the difference to discourse

As this study is based on notions of discourse, rather than truth, the task was to situate these claims about KHS's difference within an understanding of the dominant discourses[1] in which they are embedded. A basic assumption in such work is that when individuals talk about issues, they are not generally aware, at a conscious level, of the discursive origins of the notions they privilege. According to Fairclough, (1989:24) individuals internalise socially constructed and available beliefs from any number of discourses, reproducing such internalised notions in their own social practice. The power and force of such a shaping effect on society is increased by the fact that such a process is not generally apparent. Thus, the *task of this chapter* becomes one of beginning to *make apparent the underlying discourses implicit in the notions expressed by the participants with regards to KHS's difference.*

Such a descriptive discussion of discourse is considered to be not only an appropriate starting point, but also the basis for later interpretative discussions about issues of subjectivity, change and the demands of social situations. For, as Fairclough (1989:39) suggests, social subjects are constrained to operate within the subject positions set up by different discourses. Such discourses are seen as a resource for subjects, who actively and creatively combine them in ways to meet the ever-changing demands and contradictions of real social situations. A description of the significant discourses running through KHS is consequently offered as an important groundwork for understanding the interpretative analysis of the data which follows.

The major discourses running through KHS which have been isolated for discussion are those associated with Hospice, Buddhism, Spirituality and Death and Dying. The following chapters deal with each of these discourses in detail (beginning in this chapter with the hospice discourse). Also, as there were many statements by the participants which defined KHS's difference by its contrast to biomedicine's 'technological imperative', a chapter will also deal with this discourse. To start this process, this chapter will provide a summary of the participants' comments on KHS's difference and will begin to situate such 'talk' in a description of the first dominant discourse surfacing as significant in this organisation: the hospice discourse.

Affirming a difference

> We are something different and I hope that that something different stays. Because that is what energises people and sort of gives us the satisfaction (EQ).

All those interviewed clearly stated the belief that KHS was different and in significant ways. What, then, was the difference stated by those interviewed?

The comments of the participants have been interpreted as referring to two levels of difference with regards to this service. The first is at the coalface working with clients and the second is at an organisational level. This somewhat artificial, but useful, dichotomy will be maintained throughout this analysis.

When discussing work at the coalface the interviewees described KHS's difference not only by what it was, but also by what it was not. This discussion will begin with the positive statements of difference. These centered on a difference by doing, which included the notion of holism, the provision of choice, and the opportunity to die at home. This will be contrasted to the reductionist, physiological bias of mainstream medicine: a reference used by the participants to describe what KHS was not.

At the organisational level, KHS was described as a supportive, caring, and democratic organisation, which contrasted with the top down power of the hierarchical model of biomedicine.

The connecting thread which was seen to distinguish and to support this practice and organisational difference was the notion of spirituality. This description of the perception of KHS's difference as recorded in the statement of participants will now be explored in closer detail.

The difference at the coalface

> We bring a very different approach to people that we care for (EQ).

KHS is a specialist hospice service, so understandably throughout the language/texts participants defined[2] this organisations difference from other institutions working with the terminally ill (for example, tertiary care centres such as general hospitals, or primary care organisations such as community health) by its singular concern of working with the dying and their families in the community. For many participants, this shared acceptance of a common goal, expressive of this service's core values and clarity in seeing, was in itself an important aspect of this service's difference.

This difference of exclusive focus was further emphasised by a difference in practice, which incorporated notions of holism, a respect for individual choice and a comfort with and acceptance of working with the dying, underpinned by a Buddhist philosophy.

Holism

> A real comprehensiveness that is not there in some of the other organisations (EQ).

The 'talk' about KHS focused on the holistic, comprehensive, twenty-four hour service, which cared for the patient and their family from a psycho-social-physico-spiritual perspective.

The qualities underpinning the holistic approach were seen to be those of non-judgmental acceptance and compassionate, loving care. KHS reportedly attracted, and actively selected, individuals with personal strengths such as a sense of humour, an ability to work within situationally-imposed limits, integrity, compassion, warmth, a willingness to serve and an interest in self/professional development.

Such a holistic approach was seen to contain a proactive element. The anticipation of problems before a crisis occurs, backed up by the provision of extensive physical, emotional and social support, was suggested as a process which reduces carer burnout and provides the dying patient with the appropriate and necessary care. This home-based hospice service, which is respectful of alternative approaches to healing and incorporates home respite, volunteer backup and bereavement services, is seen to be so comprehensive and holistic that it was described by one interviewee as practicing 'total emersion' care.

The important contribution of volunteers

> Lots of loving commitment in the volunteers...other services don't have volunteer programs (EQ).

Volunteers were recorded as a vital aspect of such holistic care, which differentiated this service from the work of others in the metropolitian area and certainly from mainstream health services. This difference was seen to extend to the quality of person who became a volunteer, the training they received, client satisfaction with their work, the process of matching and their role description. Such volunteer backup was seen as providing the services and care which allowed KHS to holistically meet the needs of their clients. The role of the volunteers was considered to be so important in defining KHS's difference, that one interviewee stated, 'one day it will show that it is the volunteers who are making it unique'.

Karuna is choice

Central to such holistic care was a respect for choice. Protecting and supporting the individual's right to make choices, particularly in relation to their illness, was seen as a value central to the work of KHS. Such non-judgmental validation of the individual's choice was seen to contribute to the process described by the 'key word empowerment' or 'giving control back' to the individual. Such a process was seen to require sensitive support, information giving and the provision of resources as an extension of a caring and accepting relationship.

Nurses involved in this study, reflecting on their experiences elsewhere, made clear statements that this was an area of considerable difference from other places where they had been employed. Clients of KHS who were interviewed also mentioned the choice factor.

This choice factor is a very important ingredient in KHS's difference. In the words of one participant,

> Basically what I see Karuna as being is offering people a choice (EQ).

A comfort with issues of death and dying

Such a choice factor translates into attitudes about the experience of dying. Being a Buddhist based, hospice organisation, these attitudes are of central concern.

Participants made reference to the individual variability of the dying experience, and KHS's non-judgmental support of the individual's choice of how they die. Underpinning such supportive work was a stated comfort by members of this organisation with issues of death and dying. To a large degree, this comfort was attributed to the Tibetan/Buddhist philosophical foundation of the service. Such a discourse privileges ideas of rebirth, the importance of the moment of death, and the spiritual significance of the dying experience.

The opportunity to die at home

> In their own homes, they are the boss, they are in control...not close to a lot of technology and not caught up in that hype...so very empowering to be at home (EQ).

As an extension of KHS's philosophy of respecting the patient's choice is a commitment to providing the appropriate services to allow the patient the choice to die in their own home. It was stated that up to 76% of KHS's patients chose this option. Such a choice was seen as both 'precious' and 'empowering', avoiding the excessive use of technology associated with the terminal stages of life. Interviewees made it explicit that there was no expectation that to die at home was the 'right way', only that it was a unique choice offered by KHS. As has been previously mentioned, proactive steps are taken with the families of dying patients to increase their confidence and coping ability, so that this option is not too stressful.

Praxis: the difference is in the doing

The emphasis throughout the language texts is on describing KHS's difference through its praxis: the translation of ideas into practice. In the words of one participant,

> That is our strength...getting a reputation by doing (EQ).

That reputation, described by the participants as 'exemplary', was seen as a 'key' ingredient in depicting KHS's difference. Evolving by example, such a reputation was stated by those interviewed to exist at both the local, state and international level, being based on the dedication, commitment and expert knowledge of those running the service.

Difference via negitiva

> ...a very non-physical, non-physiological, non-biological kind of bias (EQ).

The idea of difference was not only described by what KHS is, but also by what it is not. Many of the participants defined KHS's difference by contrasting it with the bio-medical model. The hospital was seen to be more technology oriented, and differed on issues of environment, staffing and funding. Negative descriptives were used in relation to institutional biomedical care both for patients ('intimidating', 'disempowering') and staff ('criticising' and 'blaming').

Although KHS was seen to have incorporated some notions of the biomedical model (for example, nursing and palliative care skills, and an important role for the general practitioner), these, although acknowledged as significantly useful, were not seen as central to the role of the service.

Several statements were made to distinguish their approach from the bio-medical model's reductionist, cure oriented approach to dying, which lacked an acceptance of death. Hospital death was described as possibly painful and terrifying.

Summing up the issues at the coalface

From this discussion the description of KHS defines it to be very different to mainstream curative health organisations (where, as a later discussion of statistics will show, most people die). In the words of one participant,

> It is still unique in Brisbane, so though...(some)...are now twenty four hours a day in some areas, they don't generally have the same...they don't have the volunteers set up, they have the occasional in home respite, but they don't have the number of volunteers and they don't have the psychologists and the bereavement support and they don't have the intensity of the situation (EQ).

At the organisational level

So far, this discussion has explored the notions of KHS's difference as expressed through their work with their clients. However, as previously indicated, talk of a difference at the organisational level also surfaced in these language/texts.

A supporting environment

> (We are)...very supportive of each other in informal sense.. (EQ).

Many statements were made about the positive support for staff at KHS, describing the milieu as an accepting and loving place to be, with lots of formal and informal support structures. This was set in the context of demanding and stressful work, and contrasted to the critical and judgmental atmosphere of other health institutions. Such support was seen as essential for the emotional nourishment of workers in a caring profession.

A democratic organisation

> No layers..everyone appears to be valued evenly or equally...not ...hierarchically structured (EQ).

Participants also spoke of the considerable energy that members of KHS channelled into retaining a 'flat structure' in their organisation, where all members are valued equally, without the need for hierarchy or layers. The philosophical orientation of this organisation affirms decentralised power and seeks to meld both an egalitarian approach with an explicitly stated decision making map, so those involved feel valued but 'clear about who makes which decisions'. This was contrasted with the top down, medico-centric decision making organisation of hospitals.

A leader with a difference

> He has that specialness of Karuna...but I don't know how you are going to be putting it into words to be quite honest...that specialness and that charisma is something very deep seated...that compassion for humanity..(he) is very special...and that makes us special (EQ).

There was, however, within this organisation, one individual in particular who was acknowledged as a significant figure in describing KHS's difference and this was their 'charismatic leader'. Respectful reference was made to this spiritual leader, a Buddhist monk, whose presence was felt to place a significant and definitive stamp of difference on the KHS.

Historically, he was the key player, conceptualising and initiating the dream of this hospice project as a response to a request by his Buddhist teacher. Seen invariably as 'the spiritual leader' and linchpin of the organisation, this 'Rogerian', non-directive figure is viewed with great respect as the driving force behind this organisation. Described with superlatives, such as 'amazing', and 'wonderful', this leader's integrity is considered to be of the highest order, and his caring, compassionate commitment and dedication, is seen to be an essential ingredient in KHS's success. His genius for valuing and including quality people with highly developed and desirable professional skills has been stated by all to be the foundation stone of the organisation's growth. His special gift has been stated to lie in allowing individuals to feel they are listened to and their ideas respected. As with all charismatic leaders, their human side also alienates and in this case the interviewees also registered problems.

The connecting thread - spirituality

Whether speaking about work at the coalface or organisational issues, there was one thread which connected all the discussions, and this was the notion of spirituality.

Although it was acknowledged that the spiritual dimension was difficult to define, this aspect of KHS was perceived by all interviewed as contributing significantly to a sense of KHS's difference. In the words of one participant,

> I think to give it (spirituality) a place...to give it some sort of recognition. What I am saying is I think that is what Karuna has done (EQ).

A very generalised notion of spirituality

The language of this generalised concept of spirituality included notions of compassion, love and caring and a willingness to serve others. The Buddhist philosophy was but one discourse in this spiritual metaphysic which was stated to be a comprehensive and universal tolerance of different belief systems.

Central to the 'talk' on this spiritual essence were ideas of pure motivation, self-awareness, seen to be guiding and creating an enlightened space from which insights flows. Woven throughout the interviews were examples of such self-reflexive insight, and many participants stated that they felt that individuals embark on a spiritual journey when associated with KHS.

The spiritual link with holism

> I suppose for me it is some sense...some real sense that there is some other aspect of people than just their emotional and intellectual selves (EQ).

In terms of patient services, this spirituality was translated into a holistic understanding of the patient's needs, which included the spiritual dimension. Such a spiritual interpretation privileged existential issues, and legitimated the importance of such questions as the meaning of life and the meaning of death. The medical model, it was suggested, does not accommodate such an orientation.

The Buddhist philosophy

Karuna is also unique partly because it is a Buddhist organisation (EQ).

A distinctive difference between KHS and other similar services is the strong Buddhist influence within the organisation. Initiated by a Buddhist request, KHS is seen by many members as a Buddhist organisation. However, the language/texts described this organisation as not exclusively Buddhist, but rather, comfortably incorporating representatives from many religio-philosophical orientations. Although underpinned by a strong Buddhist spirituality, KHS is neither financially nor legally a Buddhist organisation: nevertheless, the Buddhist link is viewed as strong and significant.

Participants translated the Buddhist difference into the type of person attracted, the service provision, philosophical attitudes to dying, self-reflexivity, and a spiritual cohesion and bonding incorporating all within the organisation. Compassion, wisdom, non-harm to others, respect of difference, personal responsibility to resolve problems, and an acknowledgment of a spiritual dimension to existence were the significant Buddhist principles referred to by these interviewees.

There was a strong Eastern influence in the interpretation of these ideas of spirituality, being seen as a daily journey. KHS was described as an 'existential mirror' which confronts the individual with a reflection of their inner selves. The choice for some, it was argued, was to change or leave. Such a spiritual dimension was seen to challenge on a daily basis those involved to demonstrate caring based on pure motivation.

A concern about the fragility of the spiritual dimension

There was an explicit awareness of the description of spirituality outlined above which was valued as a fundamental ingredient in KHS's difference. Anxiety was voiced about the fragile nature of such a spiritual orientation and the steps that must be taken to preserve this core dimension of the organisation.

Beginning the translation

As has been outlined in the introduction to this chapter, the task now is to translate this stated difference to discourse. As a point of reference, such translations will be set in the context of the writings and research from the academic literature specific to each discourse.

A caveat to such discussion is that, although the different significant discourses underlying the discursive practices of KHS will be outlined separately, this does not suggest, *ipso facto,* that such discourses could be so differentiated in practice. As Fairclough states (1992:55), when pointing out the primacy of interdiscursivity and intertextuality, 'any discursive practice is defined by its relations with others, and draws upon others in *complex* ways'. There is considerable similarity and difference in the key discourses isolated for exploration in this work, as will be highlighted through the following detailed discussion.

The subsequent explorations of the different discourses are seen as the starting point, not only for understanding notions of difference but also for developing the more complex insights that arise. According to Davies, (1994:2) this is the first step in deconstruction: the location of the metaphysical and constructed nature of discursive practices or patterns of talk. Such a process seeks to ask such questions as: What are the dominant discourses privileged by these language/texts? How do the discursive practices of participants of KHS stand up to the scrutiny of the research literature on hospice/palliative care? Are there significant hospice and/or bio-medical notions being silenced? How do the notions being privileged/silenced relate to the hegemonic power base of the bio-medical model? How do the strategies of exclusion and repression advance or hinder our understanding of the work with the dying in our society? What is the core concern of Karuna's 'will to power', contained within the deconstructed centre of their discursive practices?

The commencement of this process will be the situating of KHS's hospice 'talk' in the academic writings on the palliative care/hospice discourse.

Situating hospice 'talk' in discourse

Through a discussion of the emerging literature on international discourse of hospice/palliative care, it will be shown that much of KHS's difference makes it similar to, and characteristic of, hospices world wide. It will be argued that, apart from the very significant aspect of the Buddhist discourse, the notions participants used were not very different from the hospice concepts outlined in the palliative care literature. However, the rendering of this community based, holistic hospice ideology into practice makes it different from other health organisations which work with the dying within our local culture. Such a difference in practice may reflect the slow implementation of hospice/palliative care philosophy in Australian society.

To demonstrate this similarity an overview will be provided of a range of ideas and issues commonly discussed in the hospice literature.

Elements and principles of hospice/palliative care

The term palliative care comes from the Latin *palliat* meaning cloaked or covered (Paradis, 1987:77) To palliate means to alleviate without curing: to mitigate. The focus is on comfort and symptom relief. In short, palliative care is 'care designed to alleviate pain and suffering, rather then to cure or rehabilitate' (McNulty and Holderby, 1983:12). Such care can start at the time of diagnosis, and need not be restricted to just the care of the dying.

The hospice model of care has a more definite focus, as it emphasises palliation of symptoms of incurable illness. According to the precise definition of the National Hospice Organisation (Munley, 1983:79), a hospice is 'a program of palliative and supportive services which provides physical, psychological, social and spiritual care for dying persons and their families'. Although, hospice work is predominantly with those in the final stages of a terminal illness, there are two important caveats to such a principle. Firstly, there is no necessity for mutual exclusiveness between the cure and the hospice world. As outlined by Saunders, 'the way must be kept open always for the patient to move, when appropriate, between the "cure" system of the hospital and the "care" system of the hospice, ensuring that nobody ever risks becoming locked into one or the other' (1981:93). Secondly, such an interpretation of intervention in the later stages of the dying trajectory does not legitimate a presupposition that the hospice is a place to be used 'When nothing more can be done'. Palliation is viewed as a hopeful, realistic goal (Koff, 1980), success being measured not in terms of prolongation of life gained, or tumour shrinkage, but more importantly in terms of the quality of experience and the demonstrated ability to care for the patient and their family.

Holism[3] *and democratic care*

Such care is based on the integration of a multidisciplinary plan of care, addressing the physical, spiritual, social and emotional needs of each patient and their family (Siebold, 1992:2). This comprehensive response to the individual's needs is termed holistic care.[4] Because of the holistic nature of hospice/palliative care work, it cannot be accomplished by one professional, no matter how dedicated or skilled. Such work requires a commitment to effective team work. Therefore, respecting the autonomy of fellow professionals is of great importance.

Some authors suggest that such respect for different disciplines breaks down interprofessional boundaries and necessitates a degree of role blurring which emphasises responsiveness to the patient's total needs (Munley, 1983:58). Such organisations being characterised by the collegial ('we spirited') orientation of the staff and the characteristic intimacy of staff interaction with patients and families.

However, other authors such as Vachon (1993:600) suggest that such role blurring for health professionals working within the hospice is often interpreted as role ambiguity and contributes to stress and burnout, emphasising the importance and usefulness of clear role definition and explicit description in areas of decision making responsibility.

Certainly, however, in comparison to hospitals and nursing homes, hospices are seen to be characterised by a democratic, flat organisational structure, where decisions are made by a team, with the patient and family as equal partners (Hamilton and Reid, 1980:137).

'Low-tech' pain and symptom control

In hospice care, symptom control is accomplished with the use of a minimum of diagnostic studies and invasive therapeutic measures. Furthermore, symptoms are considered to include psychosocial problems as well as physical complaints. As a result, hospice patients receive relatively little technologically, but gain a great deal of personal attention (Zimmerman, 1981:30).

In hospice care, pain control receives special attention: the hospice vision centres on reducing the distraction and fear of suffering from pain, and hence assisting the patient to think clearly and maintain significant interpersonal relationships (Mor et al., 1988:10).

As a speciality service, clinical skills are considered important in hospice care: highly skilled and knowledgeable practitioners are an essential ingredient in competent hospice care (Dobratz, 1990:116).[5]

The importance of choice

The goal of such service provision is to facilitate the exercise of control and choice by the patient and their family and to affirm at every step the individual uniqueness, based on a central value of 'respect for persons'.[6] In the words of Saunders, the founder of this movement,

> A patient should be enabled to live until he dies, at his own maximum potential, performing to the limit of his physical activity and mental capacity, with control and independence where ever possible. He should be recognised as the unique person he is, and helped to live as part of his family and in other relationships with some awareness from those around of his own hopes and expectations and of what has deepest meaning for him (Saunders, 1994).

The reference to 'meaning' in this statement can be seen to imply that hospice care has a spiritual aspect. It is argued that the very process of confronting death moves the individual into the 'realm of spirituality' (Kirschling and Pittman, 1989:1).

The 'realm of spirituality'

As an extension of the interpretation of holistic care, there is broad agreement among hospice workers that spirituality is too critical to be left to the clergy, but is shared by all involved in the care of the patient and their family (Millison and Dudley, 1992:51). The concept of spirituality is broader than religion and includes the individual's quest for meaning, either through religion or a simple existential questioning of the events of every day life. The essence of spiritual care giving is the ability to enter into the world of others and to respond with feeling (Millison and Dudley, 1992:51). The hospice definition of spirituality is concerned with promoting interpersonal bonding and respecting personal quests for meaning; it is similarly broad and individualised (Bellingham et al., 1989; Munley, 1983:229). Such a spiritual perspective is respectful of multicultural pluralism and is broad enough to cover the spiritual needs and concerns of those who do not have formal religious beliefs. As expressed by a patient, 'the fact that they are so giving and so caring to me is spiritual'(Munley, 1983:245).

The normalisation of death

Hospice care incorporates the concept of the 'normalisation of death': death is seen as a very human event, a legitimate and normal process (Hamilton and Reid, 1980:48), and an inevitable part of life. Hospice philosophy accepts that death is a fact of human existence, not to be avoided, but to be faced and accepted.

The choice of place of dying is a central principle in hospice care. The comfort and security of one's own home is considered a desirable place to die, although it is accepted that the individual may chose, because of practical considerations, pain management or lack of social support, to die in an institutional setting (Blues and Zerwekh, 1984:8).The final days and hours of death are given particular attention, with the opportunities being provided for the patient to experience the final moments in a way meaningful to them (Mor et al., 1988:10).

Family involvement

Open acceptance of death mandates that families be involved in hospice care. The family is the main care provider, as well as the recipient of hospice services of care. A foundational value of respect for the choice and wishes of the patient and his/her family necessitates that professional care providers should defer to the judgement of the patient and family (Bass, 1985:308-9). Priority is given to supporting the individual's lifestyle for as long as possible, with a respect for the individual's ethnicity, cultural orientation, social and sexual preferences, (Koff, 1980:69).

Saunders translates such broad perspective into two principles of care:

1 terminally ill person's own preferences and life-styles must be taken into account in all decision making,

2 family members and other caregivers also have legitimate needs and interest that must be taken into consideration (cited in Mor et al., 1988:9).

Bereavement follow-up

Bereavement follow-up is an essential component of hospice care (Byrd and Taylor, 1989:46) seen as an extension of the basic hospice conviction that the family as well as the patient should be seen as the unit of care (Manning, 1984:89).

To 'truly' care

Central to such a service provision is the important quality of caring. This is stressed throughout the literature. Such caring provides the individual with a sense of security and trust, and hence safety, possible only when there is a dependable plan of care maintained by people who really do care (Mor et al., 1988:10). To 'really' care, to 'truly'care is considered the important ingredient, as stated by Pratt and Filicky-Peneski, 'it must be truly caring. Caring is many things: it is a sense of humour, recognising our own feelings and dealing with them appropriately, an attitude of self-confidence and self-worth, trusting in our own intuition. Caring is a touch, it is love, it is time, it is understanding' (1983:127).

The valuable contribution of volunteers

As an extension of the philosophy of care, hospices are characterised by their effective use of volunteers (Byrd and Taylor, 1989:41; Seibold et al., 1987:43). Being variously described as the 'backbone' or the 'spirit' of the hospice movement, the volunteers offer unpaid practical, emotional and spiritual support, as additional services to the paid professionals, which enhance the care of families.[7] Volunteers are usually recruited, trained, matched, supported and supervised in their work with patients and families (Lafer, 1991:161).

The issue of equity

Equity issues are an important agenda in the provision of hospice services. Health needs, not the ability to pay, is the stated criteria of patient acceptance into hospice services (Breindel and Boyle, 1979:42; Munley, 1983:80).

The essential components

In summary the essential components of a hospice program have been outlined by the National Hospice Organisation (American), and include the following -

- family participation in care planning
- 24 hour, seven day a week availability of the hospice team
- psychosocial support and educational programming
- integrated inpatient and home care
- bereavement services after the patient's death
- use of volunteers (MacDonald, 1990).

Other authors, whilst affirming these points, also include and emphasise the necessity of skilled nursing care, with the relief of pain and distressing symptoms (Blues and Zerwekh, 1984:7), as seen by the following list of major elements in hospice care for the dying -

- Symptom control: a thorough but noninvasive assessment, individually titrated drugs regularly administered to control pain and retain alertness, and constant attention to sources and therapies for any discomfort
- Treating patient and family as a unit of care
- Available home and inpatient care, 24 hours a day, seven days a week
- Physician-directed medical services, nurse-directed nursing care, and interdisciplinary attention to the patient's physical, psychological, spiritual, and social suffering
- Volunteers to help the family maintain a normal daily life
- Continuing bereavement care for the family and support throughout mourning (Blues and Zerwekh, 1984:7).

Conclusion

Ideologically and conceptually the 'talk' of those associated with KHS reflects the theoretical frameworks of the hospice care movement.[8] In relation to such concepts, KHS's difference lies not so much at a theoretical level, but rather at the point of praxis. The genius of KHS is that it actually puts such ideas into practice.

However, these ideas were not the only notions sanctioned, with regards to difference. The next chapter continues to contextualise the language/texts of the participants to discourse, with a particular interest in examining notions associated with, but marginal to, the hospice discourse: to explore the difference within the difference!

Notes

1 The Foucaultian notion of discourse as outline in the previous chapter is used in this context.

2 The statements made by participants in this research will be referred to in past tense. This is for two reasons. Firstly, such statements were actually made previous to the writing up of this text. Secondly, to record such statements in the present tense conveys the positivist notion that such ideas are absolute or true rather than notions expressed in talk.

3 Holism is an evolving term, first coined by Smuts in 1926, which according to the research of Ham Ying (1993) should incorporate the notion of the person as a total being who is greater than the sum of the parts.

4 Pelletier describes holistic medicine as follows (1990:13) 'an orientation has emerged in health care which has been termed holistic medicine, derived from the Greek "holos" meaning "whole". Fundamental to holistic medicine is the recognition that each state of health and disease requires a

consideration of all contributing factors; psychological, psychosocial, environmental, and spiritual.'

5 A holistic approach does not exclude clinical skills. As Griffin (1993:310) explains, 'it is important to underline that holism accepts the need for swift and sophisticated medical and surgical intervention where appropriate: it does not reject technology but acts in conjunction with it.'

6 Zerwekh (1995:35) emphasises the importance of this notion when he states that encouraging Choice is so integral to hospice that all other competencies then extend as limbs from that center. Hospice nurse experts are 'absolute firm believers in letting people do it the way they want to.'

7 Patchner and Finn (1987:136) report that 'in a study of hospice services in the United States, Buckingham and Lupu found that a sample of twenty-four hospice programs, all but one involved volunteers. The programs had an average of sixty-eight volunteers, which ranged from three to 400 per hospice. Volunteers engaged in a variety of activities.'

8 In relation to hospice/palliative care, this work seeks only to situate the talk of KHS within the academic literature and in so doing to acknowledge and affirm its compatibility and similarity to hospices world wide. KHS's discourse is perceived as building on and absorbing the talk of the international hospice movement. The same cannot be said for this organisation's relationship to biomedicine, which is far more complex. Consequently, the focus for developing the interpretation will remain on KHS's relationship with biomedicine, rather than on exploring the connection between KHS and the hospice discourse.

5 Buddhism: the difference within the difference

Introducing the Buddhist discourse

> As a Buddhist based organisation the Karuna Hospice Service also acts as a compassionate service model to the dying for the world Buddhist community. Our vision springs from a Buddhist value base... (The Karuna Hospice Service Vision and Values Statement, 1995).

Clearly, Buddhist philosophy is of considerable importance to this organisation. Throughout the language/texts, such a Buddhist influence was seen to give a significant stamp of difference specific to KHS, setting it apart from other local hospice, palliative care or nursing organisations working with the dying. Consequently, such Buddhist 'talk' will be considered the second important discourse running through this service. The Buddhist 'way' of seeing, although different from the previously discussed hospice discourse, is compatible with it. Hence it is seen as the difference within the difference.

Before exploring these notions further, a few postmodern caveats need to be stated concerning the following discussion of the Buddhist discourse and its relationship to KHS.

The Buddhist element in KHS, it must be clearly understood, consists of a group of people from a Western democratic society attracted to and, for some, practitioners of, the Buddhist Eastern metaphysics. Consequently, they view such ideology through very different socialisation experiences and historical philosophical 'baggage' from an Easterner, even if matched for class, material and educational position in life, and family experience. Their 'reading' of Buddhist philosophy will be seen as interpretative texts, which reflect a Western construction of a centuries old Eastern philosophy. This does not deny, however, that a minority are serious practitioners (monk or nun) and are immersed in Buddhist culture, both locally and internationally. It also does not negate that their interpretation of Buddhist philosophy may contain many of the core ingredients privileged by such organisations as the Foundation for the

Preservation of the Mahayana Tradition (FPMT). Thus, the task is not to grade the purity of their Buddhist concepts, but rather to explore the ideas sanctioned and repressed within the participants' talk of the influence of Buddhism on KHS. The task of this chapter is not to explore the conceptual framework of Buddhism, per se, but rather to keep the focus steadily on this local, particular, organisation-specific interpretation of Buddhist beliefs, a feature, in any case, characteristic of post modern research (Seidman and Wagner, 1992:7).

Such a discussion will be situated within appropriate academic texts on Buddhism (manifest intertextuality), but only in so far as it relates to the context of the KHS. The principal questions are, 'What affirmations of reality do the language/texts on Buddhism ideologically 'fix' for the providers and recipients of this service?'; 'How are social relations produced and reproduced through the knowledge/power of Buddhist ideology?'

The following discussion focuses on the way in which the Buddhist 'talk' of participants resonates with the central concepts of Buddhism that emerge in the academic writings. Emphasis is also placed on demonstrating how these principles are compatible with an organisation devoted to community hospice care. Such a discussion seeks to provide the conceptual ground work for understanding later interpretations about the influence of Buddhist discourse on this service, both organisationally and at the coalface of KHS's work with the client.

Academic reflections on KHS's Buddhist discourse

> What is different is our spiritual philosophy is Buddhist (EQ).

Buddhism, with its 2500-years history of development, is a diverse tradition incorporating different schools of thought (Florida, 1994:105). Of the two predominant Asian schools, the Mahayana tradition, which is the dominant Buddhist discourse within Karuna, is particularly known for its tradition of tolerance and adaptation to local customs (ibid).

The Buddhist ideological influence in this organisation is an important factor influencing its stated difference. Indeed, the very name Karuna is the Buddhist word for compassion. Some participants spoke in detail of the Buddhist principles which guide their work. Even non-Buddhist members of the organisation spoke with great respect for the influence of the Buddhist philosophy and about their attraction to, and comfort with, the following Buddhist ideas.

Compassion and wisdom

Compassion (or *karuna*), and wisdom (or *prajna*), according to Florida (1994:107) are the core values in the Buddhist metaphysic, and are intricately linked together as the essence of the Buddhist way: compassion being the practical expression of wisdom (ibid). Metaphorically described as the pillars of Buddhist teaching, wisdom and compassion are seen as one (Humphreys,

1977:109): each one is considered dangerous without the other. Such a Buddhist concept of universal compassion has traditionally been tied to the care of the ill through the provision of a caring and loving service, which aims to benefit those suffering (Ratanakul, 1988:302).

The Buddhist principles articulated by the participants, although concise and without full description, were reflective of these core Buddhist principles as exemplified by the following language/text,

> I guess compassion ... they call the two wings of enlightenment wisdom and compassion... and so I guess compassion and wisdom in trying to cut through some of your own (defenses), in trying to just be more open to situations and less defensive and ego centred or more just open and not always trying to do the best for me and protect me (EQ).

A practical metaphysic

As seen by the above quote there is a direct connection between Buddhist principles and everyday personal psychology. Indeed, according to Ward (1947:61), the philosophy of Buddhism is chiefly psychological. As will be seen by the following discussion, the Buddhist metaphysic is concerned with the role of desire,[1] intention, personal behaviour,[2] wisdom, and most importantly insight.[3] Throughout the literature on Buddhism, and certainly as evidenced by the language/texts, abstractness is not privileged as a virtue by itself, as is more the case in Western philosophical theory. The Buddhist metaphysic is guided by religious insight, rather than philosophical abstract and rational argumentation. Buddhists speak of a 'religious path', a 'spiritual journey'; their philosophical orientation is pre-eminently practical (Florida, 1994:107). There is no dichotomous separation between intellect and psychology, the first step to wisdom is self-domination: 'he who conquers himself is the greatest warrior' (Humphreys, 1977:61). This idea was clearly expressed by one of the participants, when they stated that,

> Everything about Buddhism is about how you see the world...everything and so it all comes back to you (EQ).

Unlike Western thought that seeks solutions to problems through generating change in the environment, the Eastern Buddhist philosophy does not cultivate the dualistic notion of subject and object. Instead, the traditional Mahayana perspective emphasises the essential emptiness and relativity of all things (Batchelor, 1990:32).[4] To face suffering is not so much to alter the environment, but rather to cultivate an understanding of the self (or to be metaphysically more correct - the no-self) through the inner powers of self-control and self-emancipation (Crook and Fontana, 1990:15).

This is not so much a silencing of the importance of the outside world, but is rather a realisation that what we discover outside ourselves must inevitably be conditioned by (in a sense be a consequence of) what we discover inside (Fontana, 1990:43). This notion of the 'no-self' is explained by Kalupahana when he stated the view that,

> The Buddha was not prepared to posit an agent or a mental substance behind the psychological process represented by such things as feeling (*vedana*), perception (*sanna*), dispositions (*sankhara*), and consciousness (*vinnana*). 'I think, therefore I am' (*manta asmi*; cf. the cartesian *cogito ergo sum*) is a conclusion to be repudiated (1976:39).

Consequently, an inward discovery is not a journey into egoic consciousness, as in Western psychology, which privileges the importance of a sense of self or a personal identity to be protected, developed and self actualised. Rather, the Buddhist notion of the inward journey is to discover the non-self, 'the original self', which is both pure and empty: in short, to discover our Buddha-nature. Buddhism steps outside the dualism of Western thought and posits the interconnectedness of all existence which is integrated into a single, non-dual reality. This notion of the non-self, and its importance to the practical psychology of Buddhist action is summed up by Ryomin when he states,

> When the ego is emptied and one has become non-ego, that emptying bespeaks a non-duality of self and others, a state in which 'The heavens and I are one root, all things and I are one body'. At that point the sufferings of others become one's own sufferings, and a compassionate lament over the sufferings of others wells up of its own accord. This is the cry of compassion (*karuna*). Even if one becomes a Buddha, one cannot stay in *nirvana*. The vow to be a bohisattva and devote one's efforts to the salvation of the myriad of sentient beings is the natural outcome, the 'wondrous practice', of enlightenment at work (1990:86).

This Buddhist emphasis on self-investigation is a central factor in both KHS's 'difference' and 'resistance', and so will be a recurring theme in developing the interpretation of this work. Such self investigation will be interpreted as very similar to the postmodern concept of self-reflexivity, the presence of this dimension impacts on all aspects of this organisation. Whilst promoting ideas of self awareness and responsibility for one's own actions, such an idea silences the right to impose dogma and values on others, and incorporates a respect and flexibility, honesty and humility in relationships with others. This is definitely seen as a positive aspect of working in this organisation, as seen by the following statement of a participant,

> Working in a Buddhist organisation I feel more obligation or whatever at my own stuff and work through it rather than trying to find ways of externalising it...it has an incredible influence (EQ).

A flexible metaphysic with a central psycho-therapeutic message (Ross, 1993:160), moral rather than intellectual purpose (Ward, 1947:61), and practical foundation (Florida, 1994:107), Buddhist philosophy, as interpreted by members of this organisation, has something very important to offer the discipline of bioethics (ideas to be explored in a later chapter).

Tolerance

> The basic thing... I guess is tolerance, it is a religion or philosophy which sees that there are many different paths..it doesn't say this is the right way as some religions do..it can embrace all religious beliefs that don't cause harm to people (EQ).

Buddhism is documented as a tradition of tolerance, which affirms freedom in matters of belief, worship and religious practice (Florida, 1994:105). The Mahayana Buddhist psycho-philosophical view is based on the principle that no one has the right to impose his or her beliefs on another person (Dalai Lama, 1995:1). To understand such tolerance it is necessary to have some appreciation of the Buddhist construction (or it could be argued deconstruction) of the notion of reality. Such ideas do not easily lend themselves to literary descriptions, belonging more comfortably to the experiential dimension of human spiritual comprehension. Indeed, the training to develop insight through Buddhist metaphysics is through direct contact with the non-discursive basis of mind, through methods that deconceptualise the processes of experience (Crook, 1990:93).

According to Florida (1994:107), Buddhist notions of reality privilege ideas of 'flux' and 'interconnectedness', where all in our world exist in relation to everything else that exists: unsubstantial sentient beings in a constant state of flux, in temporary, contingent relationships with similar beings. The only absolute truth is emptiness. These ideas are clearly expressed by Crook and Fontana, when they write,

> This flux, the unending relationship of cause and effect operating in time, is the basis for what he called the 'principle of interdependent origination'. All things are empty of self-nature (anatta), everything is nothing other than the process which is the expression of this principle. The Void of Buddhism is thus not non-existence, but rather the absence of discrete entitiveness in a cosmic flow of energy (1990:3).

Hence, Buddhism is ultimately a viewpoint of relativism, incorporating beliefs in the essential emptiness and relativity of all things (Batchelor, 1990:32).

Simplisticly stated according to Buddhist philosophy, reality is not something that the individual discovers outside themselves, 'out there', but rather it is an inward journey, something carried with the individual throughout life, waiting to be realised.

As has previously been discussed, the Buddhist approach is a practical one, expressed in the notion of a spiritual path or journey. This practical metaphysic is directly related to the notion of tolerance. 'Right view' and 'right action' are not sustained by faith or by the dictates of those in authority, but rather by the psychological rewards of unselfish living/selfish giving, through the virtues of compassion and wisdom. It is a spiritual path that affirms the importance of 'seeing the Christ in everyone' (to mix a metaphor) and of loving one's neighbour as oneself. Such giving is, quite simply, the natural thing to do: there is no element of sacrifice, of do-gooding, or of obedience to an external moral code. It is a practical metaphysic, which views love, compassion, and the unity of all things as true, and hatred, dissension, and division as being false. According to this philosophy, the way to realise this truth is by our actions ('right action') not simply to 'know' it with our minds. This 'view' must then be translated through the way life is lived into 'right action': a seeking to purify the mind by loving and compassionate behaviour to all living beings, rejecting pride, status, selfishness, defensiveness, aggression, and immorality. Love and tolerance of others, as an essential ingredient in Buddhist philosophy, are intricately linked with the individual's spiritual path. To practice such tolerance is an act of being wisely selfish (Crook and Fontana, 1990). Simply stated, in the words of one interviewee,

> (It is a)...basic principle of Buddhism that...that caring for others is a source of happiness and that if you are self-centred and care only about yourself that is a cause for sadness. So actually, the two things go hand in hand: your own happiness, your own satisfaction and being of service to others. It is what the Dalai Lama calls being wisely selfish. If you can generate compassion and kindness towards others you will have your own happiness (EQ).

Such a caring, compassionate tolerance of others in the language/texts of the KHS is not just privileged in relation to the families they care for, but also in relation to the members of the organisation and the wider social network. As with the previously mentioned notion of self-investigation, this virtue of tolerance emerges as one of central importance, both in defining 'difference' and in understanding 'resistance'. Already mentioned in the discusion on hospice philosophy, this notion is a recurring theme and will be dealt with in depth on the section on 'resistance'. It will suffice at this point to state that caring, compassionate tolerance is a significant spiritual notion privileged in the discursive practices of this organisation, and one which impacts on the creation of difference and the negotiation of resistance for KHS.

The duty to do no harm

Another Buddhist notion is similar to the bioethical principle of non-maleficence, or 'above all else do no harm' (Johnstone, 1994:92). As stated by one participant,

> Dalai Lama says the basic foundation is if you can't do anything else, don't do any harm to anybody (EQ).

The Buddhist duty to do no harm, called *ahimsa*, is seen as important in human relationships in general, but especially in medicine (Florida, 1994:110), where one is dealing with the vulnerable, those already experiencing the harm of pain and helplessness, of disease, disability and dying. Ratanakul, who has researched and published on Buddhist bioethics, describes the principle of non-harm as a fundamental rule in Eastern health care. According to the central Buddhist spiritual ideal of loving service, the primary concern of the health care professional (as in the West), ought to be the well-being of the patient only, and should include a concern to above all else do no harm (1986:2-3). Indeed, the duty of *ahimsa,* when applied to those suffering from illness that cannot be cured, parallels conceptually with our Western ideas on palliative care. The idea being to 'cloak', alleviate, or lessen the distress, expressed by Ratanakul as, 'if one cannot remove it (harm or disease), our duty is to alleviate it, lessen it (i.e. relieve the suffering, care for and comfort the dying and maintain as best we can those beyond our capacity to cure)' (1986:99).

The significance of death

As can be seen by such notions as *ahimsa, karuna, and prajna,* there is a great similarity and compatibility between the Buddhist discourse and that of hospice/palliative care. Central to both discourses are not just beneficence, compassion and wisdom, but a belief in the significance of the dignity and importance of dying. There is difference within this similarity, however, as will be seen by the following discussion on the significance of the moment of death.

> Having studied the Tibetan literature on death and dying and personally I am totally convinced that the amazing understanding that the Tibetan understanding of dying can make (EQ).

Tibetan Buddhism is a metaphysic which points to an understanding of the significance of death, as an essential ingredient in understanding the meaning of life. In an organisation dealing mainly with the dying, the language/texts understandably reveal many elements of the Tibetan Buddhist discourse on dying.

The idea that death is 'extremely significant', or indeed, the 'culmination of all life', and hence, the moment of death is the 'most important moment in your life', is similar in many ways to the hospice concept of death-with-dignity, although it offers much more than a respect for the dying person. The intense significance flows from the Buddhist idea of reincarnation. A calm and peaceful death can positively improve the next rebirth (or *samsara*), despite negative *karma* of past lives. As stated by Rinbochay and Hopkins,

> At the time of death attitudes of long familiarity usually take precedence and direct the rebirth. For this same reason, strong attachment is generated for the self, since one fears that one's self is becoming nonexistent. This attachment serves as the connecting link to the intermediate state between lives, the liking for a body in turn acts as a cause establishing the body of the intermediate (*bardo*) being (1985:9).

According to Rinpoche (1992:224), such a privileging of the significance of the moment of death, is predicated on the assumption that the last thought and emotion that the individual has before death has an extremely powerful determining effect on their immediate future, their rebirth into a new life. Such ideas were clearly articulated by some of the research participants who made such statements as,

> In terms of understanding death and dying and understanding all aspects of dying, Buddhism has a vast knowledge and a huge amount of knowledge of that whole process and it helps people with that process in understanding how to make the most of that experience. There is an enormous spiritual opportunity at death and the spiritual practitioners can become liberated and enlightened at the time of death. The person is able to physically transfer their consciousness to a purer state, to go beyond suffering in this existence (EQ).

> In Buddhist teaching there is a lot of emphasis on existential issues, the meaning of life, redirecting your life to have meaningful experiences in life and death (EQ).

Interestingly, although this doctrine of *samsara,* (or rebirth) is linked closely with the Buddhist law of *karma* (Fernando, 1985:37), an understanding and respect for which is the primary *modus operandi* of the Buddhist spiritual path, participants made no mention of the word *karma* during the interviews. Described as a moral or ethical value (ibid), *karma* is a popularly understood concept in Western culture, and so its silencing from these texts may or may not be of significance. This certainly could be one of the many questions arising from these findings that could lead to further research. As the previously stated focus of this chapter is to situate the KHS discourse on Buddhism within the literary texts, not to explore Buddhism in full, these ideas will not be elaborated further.

A willingness to serve

In translating the Buddhist philosophy into the practical path of compassionate action, ideals of being in service to others, and avoiding the pitfalls of being self-serving are sanctioned as fundamental practical virtues. In the words of one of the participants,

> How Buddhist principles translate with Karuna, is very much in terms of service delivery, in that we are trying to fulfil the needs of the other person...we are not here to be self-serving...the whole organisation is customer driven (EQ).

The desire to serve is seen in Buddhist literature as the moral imperative of compassion (Florida, 1994:107): a self-giving, self-denying act of generosity of spirit. Ratanakul states, to demonstrate by example, 'when nurses or doctors stay with patients who need them, night and day, foregoing rest and family, this is an act of compassion, of self-denial' (1988:312).

This aspiration to be of benefit to all living things is described in the Mahayana Buddhist literature as a desire directing the central path to Buddhahood (Dalai Lama, 1995:10). As has been demonstrated by the provision of language/texts, such a desire is privileged throughout the discourse of this organisation. One such example being,

> Buddhist principles of serving others, the whole organisation was based on what the client needs, what do they and their family need, and how can we meet it (EQ).

Conclusion

As can be seen by this discussion, the language/texts which privileged Buddhist ideas sit clearly and demonstrably within the recorded literary discourse on this Eastern philosophy, and complement and affirm many of the ideals from the discourse on hospice/palliative care.

As compatible as hospice notions are with Buddhism, however, the incorporation of such a Buddhist philosophy makes KHS very different from most Western hospices recorded in the literature. Buddhism can thus be seen as the 'difference within the difference': a spiritually very different basis for hospice (which is also considered different from the mainstream way of working with the dying). This difference (Buddhist spirituality) will emerge in the analysis as both a possible obstacle to KHS's genesis (Chapter 9) and a protection against the dehumanising influence of mainstream bureaucratisation and professionalisation (Chapters 10 to 12).

Yet it will suffice at this stage in the description, to acknowledge that KHS's stated difference is situated clearly at the crossroads of two compatible and complementary discourses (hospice and Buddhism). These discourses sanction compassionate non-judgemental caring, translated into practical, loving action. As one participant clearly expressed the connection,

> Just in the day to day working with people I think that the universal care and compassion certainly comes over...there is a lot of it in palliative care. There is a lot of universal love and compassion..in itself it is not unique but it is a very supportive environment to work in I think (EQ).

Notes

1 On the issue of desire Ch'en states (1968:41) that 'to the Buddhist..suffering which is universal is caused by craving...The Buddhist discipline is directed toward the destruction of this craving, so that there is no more craving for existence, sensual pleasures, or power, and consequently no more generation of karma.'

2 As suggested in Paige and Gilliatt (1991:94) appropriate Buddhist behaviour follows the notion that 'a Buddhist who understands thoroughly

the doctrine of no-self does not put himself into antagonistic relationships with others, nor does he enter into disputes with other people. This explains his balanced and serene attitude, standing above board, leaving behind all victory and defeat. The Buddhist considers it of utmost priority to be victorious over greed, anger and delusion which are still dormant.'

3 As Ch'en (1968:41) explains, 'to have insight into things as they really are means to hold to the right view of things, which to the Buddhists consists of three fundamental truths; all existence is suffering, all existence is transitory or impermanent, and there is no permanent self or soul'.

4 Reynolds (1978:234) explains that 'in the Mahayana tradition there is a significant shift in emphasis, and the basic distinction becomes primarily epistemological; through an insight into the truth that all reality is self-less and void one realises that in the final analysis Nirvana and the cycle of transmigration (including death) are one and the same and cannot be distinguished. When this insight is fully appropriated, death is conquered and true release is experienced.'

6 Connecting the discourses: spirituality

> The Greeks understood the mysterious power of the hidden side of things. They bequeathed to us one of the most beautiful words in our language - the word 'enthusiasm' - *en theos* - a god within. Happy is he who bears a god within, and who obeys it (Pasteur cited in, Koestler, 1967:190).

To reiterate, the language texts have been situated in the context of both the palliative care/hospice and the Buddhist discourses. As central and important as this Buddhist-cum-Hospice discourse is to KHS, it shares primacy with another discourse, that of spirituality. Throughout the language/texts there arose a clearly articulated generic notion of spirituality which not only incorporated and connected ideas privileged in these other discourses, but which simultaneously embraced a well defined 'talk' of difference. A comprehension of this spiritual discourse, which will be outlined in this chapter, is central to understanding the body of interpretative findings that follow this descriptive introduction. Indeed, this *spiritual discourse of KHS, is interpreted as THE cardinal dynamic underpinning and energising this organisation's 'difference' and 'resistance' to biomedicine.*

The postmodern lens will now focus on this discourse of spirituality, which, it will be argued, is not only an important link between these other discourses, but emerges as a significant aspect of 'the way' KHS engages in its work with the dying. As will be demonstrated, the spiritual 'talk' of this organisation is central and important, both organisationally and at the coalface of patient care.

The Karuna discourse on spirituality

As with the previous deliberation on Buddhism, this discussion of spirituality is set in the context of writings related directly to the notions privileged by the language/texts. The purpose of this section is a descriptive exploration of the spiritual discourse of KHS, it is not a discussion of spirituality, per se. Such a description will then be the baseline for the later effort of interpretative understanding of the social practice of KHS. It will be argued that the aspects of KHS's particular metaphysic of spirituality not only impacts on every aspect of the relationships both within and outside this organisation, but also can be seen as having a great deal to contribute to our understanding of issues in bioethics.

The elusive dimension

Permeating the language/texts are references to the notion of spirituality. Such references were not couched in dogma, but were offered with an understanding of the difficulty of defining such a dimension, as seen by the uncertainty of definition evident in the following comments,

> I guess I still can't define that... (EQ).

> very hard to translate into research... (EQ).

> Spirituality can be a very waffly word and I think what we have tried to do is to say that...just because it is a waffly word and it might be difficult for Western culture to deal with, it doesn't mean we should leave it out (EQ).

The academic writings on spirituality acknowledge the difficulty of articulating a sufficiently comprehensive and inclusive conceptual understanding of this elusive dimension of life (Campbell, 1970:19).[1] Such definitions, when stated, often have the notions of meaning-making, transcendence, and finding love and hope as the central components.

Meaning making?

According to Kearsley, 'Spirituality can be defined as the acquisition of a belief system which serves to give meaning and purpose to one's existence' (1993:4). Frankl (1973:x), inscribes such a 'will-to-meaning' as an essential existential ingredient in human life. Along with responsibility and freedom, spiritual meaning making, Frankl believes, characterises human existence (1973:xviii). The language/texts affirm meaning-making, and the need to understand the meaning of life through the meaning of death as an important dimension of spirituality,

> What we are talking about here is actually not really what is the meaning of life, it is actually what is the meaning of death and the whole thing about death is it is a mystery and we don't know.

This desire to 'make sense' of life situations is also seen as the key ingredient in the definition of spirituality within the hospice literature, particularly when it is related to issues of suffering and death (Saunders, 1981a:7).[2]

Or holism?

In the nursing literature, this definition of spirituality as meaning-making (Burnard, 1988:36; Taylor and Ferszt, 1990:32) is often broadened out to include a holistic orientation to the patient. This can be seen by the following quote by Clark and associates (1991:68),

> Spiritual well-being, the integrating aspect of human wholeness, is characterised by meaning and hope..spiritual needs as meaning and purpose, love, trust, hope, forgiveness, and creativity.

Such an orientation includes a spiritual dimension to the physio-psycho-social understanding of the individual. Authors such as Tournier (1965) would argue that to know and relate to the whole person, one would need to know this spiritual 'reality'.[3] Spirituality, so perceived, is a 'unifying force or vital principle of a person that integrates all other dimensions of the human being' (Nagai-Jacobson and Burkhardt, 1989:19).[4] In the words of one participant, the holistic dimension to spirituality is, 'acknowledging that it is a part of their whole person' and' if we leave that out (spirituality) we leave out the most essential part of life'.

Inclusive of but different from religion

Throughout the literature, associated with such interpretations of spirituality (i.e. meaning making and holism), is a concern to make a clear distinction between the spiritual dimension and the concept of religion (Emblen, 1992; Labun, 1988:314; Millison and Dudley, 1990:65). Reversing the popularly understood belief in the interchangeability of the religion/spirituality nexus, authors see religious practices, as one *modus operandi* for expressing spiritual beliefs,[5] rather than as the only form of spirituality. As Barnard (1988:398) so clearly states,

> Spirituality is not simply participation in organized religions - though that is often one of its most significant forms of expression - but most of all it is the pursuit of meaning, of an intimation of purpose, and the sense of vital connection to one's ultimate environment. I do not take spirituality, or the search for meaning and connection, to be one part of life split off from all the rest.

Religion is but one possible component of the individual's spirituality, which is defined as that 'which touches the core of one's being where the search for personal meaning takes place...that moment when a person is seeking unconditional love, forgiveness, hope, faith, affirmation, or meaning in life' (Charnes and Moore, 1992:65). Religion consists of the commonly held beliefs, rituals, and observances that may be but one component of spirituality (ibid). Such a 'difference' between religion and spirituality is emphasised in this research where the discourse on Buddhism is included in, but treated separately to, the discourse on spirituality. Stuart and associates clearly articulate this dichotomy between religion and spirituality when they state,

> Spirituality involves the personal quest to find meaning and purpose in life and a relationship to the Mystery/Divine in the universe, *which can transcend a religious denominational connotation* (Author's emphasis, 1989:37).

The question of transcendence [6]

Central to both concepts, however, is the notion of transcendence: the individual's relationship with a higher being/reality that goes beyond anything experienced in the material world (Forbis, 1988:158; Labun, 1988:314; Smith et al., 1993:91). Such transcendence need not necessarily reflect the totalising thought of a religion, but may include an often unexamined, existential framework of day to day assumptions about a view of reality. Such an existential understanding would focus on giving and receiving love, experiencing hope, and finding meaning in life, sickness, and death (ibid). The individual's spiritual dimension is a distinct view of reality with its own network of meanings, which transcends and unifies the biological, psychological, and cultural dimensions: it makes it possible for the person to function with meaningful identity and purpose (Brooke, 1987:194).

A minimalist starting point

The literature thus reflects a questioning search for a descriptive articulation of this elusive dimension of spirituality. Hoyman's short and concise expression of this notion would at least provide a minimalist starting point for this discussion. She summarises the above discussion when sheemphasises, 'the totality of a person and recognised spirituality as that which gives life meaning and purpose.' (cited in Banks et al., 1992:221)

These two transcendent dimensions of holism and meaning making underpin the understanding of spirituality, as used in this work. Understandably in work with the dying, such a spiritual dimension takes on a central role. Indeed, it is recorded by Wald that leaders in hospice philosophy and care have been at the forefront of the quest for definition and understanding of the spiritual dimension (cited in Kaczorowski, 1989:105). This again highlights the close link between the three discourses of this organisation: hospice/palliative care, spirituality, and Buddhism. All three are normative, psycho-philosophical discourses explicitly concerned with articulating ethical responses to speculations on the mysteries of life and death.

From uncertainty to openness

So far, participants' expressions of the elusive and uncertain nature of the definition of spirituality have been situated within the academic writings on this issue. It is proposed that by silencing a definitional certainty, the notion of spirituality used in KHS's discourse is also, more importantly, privileging a theological/metaphysical openness. The tolerance of a multiplicity of perspectives has already been shown to be a central characteristic of Buddhism, but here refers to the varied voices within the language/texts, (Buddhist and non-Buddhist, Christian, Zen, atheistic) that make references to a generic spirituality. The spirituality inscribed in KHS's discourse is not one based on a singular, monotheistic dogma (postmodernist theory would refer to an absolutist grand theory of religion), but rather gives primacy to a respect for a multiplicity of perspectives and humility in knowing. Such a discourse inscribes a humble seeking of and wonderment about the possibility of 'truth', not a knowing pronunciation of any one absolute perspective, as seen by the following statements,

> I don't think it really matters what the name you put on that...it's just spirituality and I think that is proof that the different beliefs of all the people who have put in the tolerance of that (EQ).
>
> There is still a sense of it in the atheist, of the spiritual aspect, they might not be able to label it (EQ).
>
> I am not a Christian, and I am not a Buddhist...not religious as such no...I would like to think there was an element of spiritual dimension to my being. I guess I still can't define that and say that is what I am (EQ).
>
> Each of the people in the original group had their own spiritual belief, they weren't all the same and they weren't all Buddhist...it was the spiritual aspect rather than the particular Buddhist aspect (EQ).
>
> People of all different religious backgrounds but who have spiritual yearning for some sort of satisfaction (EQ).
>
> I follow no particular religious path...I could quite easily follow any (EQ).

The inscription of tolerance, respect for multiplicity, and demonstration of religious principle by constructive works rather than dogma, in a discourse that privileges the central importance of a spiritual dimension, are cardinal notions in the discourse of Karuna. Such notions impact on both aspects of difference and resistance and, it will be argued in chapter 13, have important insights to contribute to the bioethical concerns about resolving ethical issues in a pluralistic, multicultural, liberal-democratic society.

Giving spirituality a place

> They know that there is another aspect in the human mind other than the intellectual or emotional aspect. I see that as being its (Karuna's) primary uniqueness (EQ).

This discourse inscribes the legitimacy of a spiritual dimension. Statements such as the above are made with reference to a spiritual dimension, not within the context of a secular ideology. Such a discourse privileges a right to philosophical reflection, and silences the secular, materialistic interpretation of reality. The discursive practices of KHS provide a medium for reflection on a transcendent reality (/realities), the meaning of life and death, and the existential issues of daily living, interconnectedness, love, compassion and commitment. In so doing, it permits a spiritually informed subjectivity and space for action. As one participant stated,

> So I think what Karuna has done is to put it on the agenda, to give it (spirituality) some acknowledgment and say this is an important factor (EQ).

This acknowledgment of, and importance given to, the spiritual dimension by KHS, as reflected in this organisation's discursive practices is one of the most important findings of this research. As the present discussion is descriptive rather than interpretative, such significance will be left to a later section. At this point it will suffice to continue to situate the KHS discourse on spirituality within the academic writings.

Karuna style spirituality - a willingness to serve

Although a prescriptive, dogmatic definition of spirituality is silenced within these language/texts, there are innumerable examples of a multifactorial recognition of the spiritual dimension in action. The spiritual dimension is described and inscribed by action and attitude. One such action/attitude mentioned is the willingness to serve.

> A selfless motivation...willing to serve others (EQ).
>
> Incredible satisfaction at a spiritual level and an emotional level knowing that what we were doing was serving people... (EQ).
>
> ...has to do with commitment to be of service to others to be of benefit to others, so that is what I mean by spirituality. It is a genuine wish for giving service to others and not doing for your own ends (EQ).

As has been previously detailed, such an action/attitude is inscribed in this spiritual discourse through Buddhist ideology. The desire to serve, however, is also intrinsic to hospice philosophy, expressed as a multidisciplinary program of providing palliative and supportive services for the physical, psychological, social and spiritual care for dying persons and their families (Munley, 1983:79). Much has been written of the attraction of dedicated, committed, hard working, altruistic individuals to this work. Such a spiritual commitment and joy in serving others, in these language texts, is not just a principle of hospice service provision, but is a more generic motivation to be of universal benefit to humankind. The hospice is but one instrument used in the quest for this end. Such a spiritual attitude privileges self-actualisation through interconnectedness and altruism and silences the Western preoccupation with ego-need fulfilment.

Interesting research questions that would arise are: To what degree does such a discourse on spirituality marginalise the useful expression of individual needs and wants? How acceptable or legitimate is it in such a discourse to signal personal needs, ego desires, and personal motivations? Are the needs of the individual care provider silenced by privileging service to others? Is there a judgemental organisational attitude which privileges work over play, the public over the private, the other over the self? A beginning to exploring such questions will be seen in the interpretative section, although many of these questions require further research, as can be seen by the discussion in the final chapter.

A spirituality named compassion

Karuna, it has already been stated, is the sanskrit word for compassion. Understandably, nurturing the quality of compassion is an essential, stated component of this organisation's discourse on spirituality, as outlined previously. It is relevant, however, that such a concern for compassion is not just an expression of the Buddhist philosophy within this organisation, as seen by the following language texts,

> A lot of us were different religions, and different belief systems but were basically all with the same idea about compassion (EQ).
>
> He could have been a Taoist or anything..the part that interested me was the concern and the caring for others (EQ).
>
> It doesn't matter the kind of spiritual background people are as long as they have those qualities of Karuna (EQ).
>
> Basic philosophy of Karuna is to offer compassionate service and so that accommodates people from all backgrounds (EQ).

The spiritual discourse at KHS has input from many different religio-philosophical traditions, but there is a shared centre which tolerates and welcomes such difference, whilst privileging similarity of core concepts. Compassion is one such core component, inscribed as love, concern and caring kindness.[7]

And pure motivation

The notion of 'pure motivation' is also privileged within this spiritual discourse. The criterion for such motivation is the 'selfless' service to others. This idea resonates with the Buddhist practical philosophy of life essentially being a spiritual journey, where the individual seeks to engage in 'right action' through the purification of the mind by loving and compassionate behaviour to all living beings (Crook and Fontana, 1990). Easily recognisable as a key Buddhist concept, such a notion of 'pure motivation' is not as obviously privileged in the palliative care/hospice literature. 'Self awareness' would be the parallel concept, and is usually referred to in relation to understanding attitudes to death, and working with the dying (Manning, 1984:71). Although the palliative care/hospice literature is full of sensitive insights into the experience of the dying and their carers, this is not usually inscribed with an emphasis on the role of self-awareness, or the need for 'pure motivation' in acting out this sensitivity. Indeed, even within such a specific and all embracing document on spirituality as the document titled *Assumptions and Principles of Spiritual Care,* developed by the Spiritual Care Work Group of the International Work Group on Death, Dying and Bereavement (1990:75-81), no direct reference is made to self awareness or the need for purity of motivation, in spite of the sensitivity of the document to the needs of the dying.

An everyday kind of spirituality

This discourse not only offers a legitimacy to the spiritual dimension, but also provides space for the action/attitudes which it inscribes to be an integral everyday experience, as seen by one participant's statement that, 'our spirituality, to be part of our everyday life is just normal.'

Although, as already acknowledged, the practical, daily exploration of spirituality is a Buddhist concept (Florida, 1994:107), such ideas were affirmed in this organisation by both Buddhist and non-Buddhist alike. In the literature, such a notion is similar to Buber's Christian notion of the 'I and Thou', when he states,

> In every sphere, through everything that becomes present to us, we gaze toward the train of eternal You; in each we perceive a breath of it; in every You we address the eternal You, in every sphere according to its manner (1970:57).

Similarly, in the literature on Zen, the experience of enlightenment, called *satori,* is not restricted to the realm of the mystical, but, in the words of Joshu, 'Zen is your everyday thought' (cited in Fromm et al., 1960:115). According to Suzuki (1960:115-6), the Zen metaphysic focuses the process of enlightenment on the daily reality outside and inside the individual, through an open and responsive attitude to the world.

The discursive practices of KHS are a meld of at least three stated religio-philosophical traditions, these being Buddhism, Christianity, and the Zen tradition. The privileging of the importance of the daily practice of spirituality is a notion compatible with, and affirmed by, all perspectives.

A gentle spirituality

Individual interviewees stated that Karuna was the place of choice for work because of the respect for this spiritual dimension, as seen by the following statement,

> I came because it was an opportunity for me to integrate my spiritual beliefs with my work that was the reason I took the job (EQ).

Such a spirituality was seen as non-proselytising,

> We don't force it on to people but we offer the opportunity to talk about spiritual things if a person so wishes (EQ).

and privileges a gentleness,

> I suppose filtering people who have a gentle spirituality, you feel that is the ingredient that will protect the uniqueness of what Karuna is on about (EQ).

The word 'gentleness' suggests positive ideas of respect for others, the ability to listen rather than impose, and an ability to flex rather than confront. At the same time, however, if set in the context of other ideas sanctioned by this discourse, such as service to others, pure/selfless motivation, it could also be silencing an acknowledgment of strong feelings, a forum for the honest discussion of difficult issues, or the individual's right to express negative emotions. This discourse is certainly influenced by Eastern ideas, which suggest the limitations of egoic consciousness (i.e. the 'I', 'me', 'mine' consciousness) articulating problems caused by over-identity with the local, conditioned 'self' (Ross, 1993:167). This is amply demonstrated by Ross (1993:169), when she discusses the Buddhist strategy for handling the vicissitudes of life,

> You learn to sit still and endure gross discomfort with equanimity. This learning process manifests psychologically. The experience becomes a metaphor for living. Your learn at a deep level to meet adversity in the course of the day with equanimity, with a 'this too will pass' mentality. In other words, you don't feed egoic consciousness and karmic reactions by constantly getting caught up in problems. In the words of the Persian poet Anwari Soheili:
> *If thou has lost possession of a world,*
> *Be not distressed, for it is nought;*
> *Or hast thou gained possession of a world,*
> *Be not o'erjoyed, for it is nought.*
> *Our pains, our gains, all pass away:*
> *Get thee beyond the world, for it is nought*
> (quoted in Wei, 1982:117).

Such ideas could privilege a controlled, selfless personality, marginalising an emotional, self-expressive reaction to problems.

However, although selfless dedication is sanctioned in this discourse, that does not mean, *ipso facto*, that there was no expressed awareness of the individual needs being met through such a purist motivation. Throughout the language/texts there was ample evidence of what postmodern theorists would call self-reflexivity: an awareness of one's own discourse.[8] Although this will be discussed in more detail later, it is important to note here that such reflexivity was demonstrated in relation to the spiritual discourse, as seen by the following text,

> I think for the first couple of years we needed that reward...because times were very difficult at times, and so we had to be getting something out of it to keep going, and what we were getting is incredible satisfaction at a spiritual level (EQ).

In summary

The chapter has centred on a discussion of the ideas privileged in the language/texts of KHS regarding its discourse on spirituality. The expression of such ideas at the coalface with clients is reflective of the holistic concept of hospice. Distinct from the emotional and intellectual level, spirituality was seen as an essential part of life and integral to KHS's work with clients. Such spiritual care was seen as the responsibility of all team members. This philosophy of holistic care, involving a team of caring individuals, resonates throughout the literature on palliative care/hospice (Corr and Corr, 1983:4; Clark, 1993:23; Manning, 1984:14; Seibold, 1992:2).

Individual participants also spoke of their own individual spiritual journey, which helped them to understand the spiritual dimension, prepared them for the work, or gave them real grief when they had to leave the organisation. The idea of a personal journey is a central concept in much of the literature on spirituality (Ross, 1993; Fromm et al., 1974; Crook and Fontana, 1990; Campbell, 1988). Such notions affirm the individual's natural connection with the inner realms, and a transcendent reality, silencing what has been described as the 'impoverishment of atheistic materialism' which, by definition, only concerns itself with what is measurable and observable (Ross, 1993:239).

As many of the ideas on the hospice-spirituality continuum are statements of notions silenced in the bio-medical model, a full appreciation of this discourse will be delayed until it can be contextualised within a discussion of the values and assumptions underpinning biomedicine (the task of chapter 8). At this stage, it is important to note that KHS's spiritual discourse will be interpreted and presented not only as a vital factor in this organisation's difference, but also (as the discussions in later chapters will show) as a significant dynamic in maintaining KHS's vision of implementing holistic care in the face of mounting pressure to move to bureaucracy and professionalism by mainstream hegemonic forces. In short, a comprehension of the importance of KHS's spiritual discourse is central to understanding the assumptions on which the interpretation of this research is developed.

This discussion has situated KHS's discourse on spirituality within the academic literature. KHS's spiritual discourse has been highlighted as a cardinal factor in understanding the development of the analysis, and its relationship to biomedicine has been introduced. To continue to build on this examination of KHS's difference, the already mentioned notions arising out of the hospice-cum-Buddhist spiritual discourse will now be set within the emerging discourse on death and dying.

Notes

1 Ross who undertook doctoral studies on the topic of spirituality acknowledges the 'plethora' of definitions but settles on three important components of spirituality, these being, a. meaning, purpose and fulfilment b. hope/will to live c. belief and faith in self, others and God (1994). Such a schema will be used although the concept of God will be replaced by the notion of transcendence.

2 According to Fife (1994:309) 'the concept of meaning commonly refers to the relationship between individuals and their world, as well as to individual's unique perceptions of their place within that world'. It is the construction of this relationship of meaning which is a central aspect of adaption during serious illness (ibid).

3 Such a definition of spirituality does not remove it from the realm of everyday experience but rather as Stiles explains (1990:235) 'the spiritual is not elusive or hidden behind or beyond experience. Rather, transforming, transcending moments are part of human experience and can be described and shared. Knowing the spiritual is to know one's self, others, and a transcendent dimension of experience.'

4 Stuart and associates (1989:36) describe this holistic dimension of spirituality when they write, 'spiritual well-being can be seen as a cornerstone of health, enabling holistic integration of one's inner resources, the often compartmentalised facets of the physical body, rational mind, emotional psyche, and intuitive spirit.'

5 Emblen's research (1992:41) has shown that in definitions of religion, six words appear most frequently and these are system, beliefs, organized, person, worship, practices; whilst in definitions of spirituality nine words appear most frequently being, personal, life, principle, animator, being, God (god), quality, relationship, transcendent. Only the word person (al) appeared on both lists. Emblen states, 'it was concluded that spirituality is currently the broader term and may subsume aspects of religion.' Indeed the research of Taylor and associates (1994:486) suggests a problematic relationship between religion and spirituality when they state that 'it is possible that a high degree of religiosity can contribute to a nurse having difficulty appreciating the spiritual well-being of a patient who believes differently. In addition, the very religious nurse may be inappropriately

eager to proselytise.'

6 Emblen (1992:46) suggests that it was the addition of holism and humanism which gradually changed the way nurses viewed the religious and the spiritual to include broader terms such as transcendence.

7 In an exploration of nurse-family spiritual relationships Stiles (1990) documented the caring orientation of 'being with' rather than 'doing to' as central to the affirmation of a spiritual dimension, which according to Stiles's research is revealed through the development of caring relationships.

8 This notion which arises out of the literature on discourse (Davies, 1994:19) refers to the the individual's ability to step outside the 'reality' constituted by their own 'talk', will be discussed in chapter 9.

7 A changing discourse: death and dying

> The classical deathbed scene, with its loving partings and solemn last words, is practically a thing of the past; in its stead is a sedated, comatose, betubed object, manipulated and subconscious, if not subhuman (Fletcher cited in Stoddard, 1979:107).

KHS is a hospice organisation whose aim is 'to provide the highest quality service to people with terminal illnesses and their loved ones from the time of diagnosis through the bereavement period' (Vision and Values Statement). Its work is situated at the coalface of death and dying within our community. As has already been discussed, several discourses inscribe the rationale for this work with the terminally ill, these being hospice/palliative care, Buddhism, spirituality and, very marginally, the Biomedical discourse. Each of these discourses is, in turn, inscribed and silenced by the more generic, modern, Western discourse on death and dying in our society. A full understanding of the research findings on KHS's 'difference' requires, it is suggested, the contextualising of the results to the more generic and changing discourse on death. Such an elaboration extends the ongoing theme that *different discourses translate into different 'ways' of responding to issues of death and dying*. Also, such a discussion is vital in setting the stage for the second analytic task of this work - an examination of KHS's resistance to the hegemony of mainstream health.

The art of dying: an historical perspective

In pre-modern, Western societies, death was not individualised and primarily personal, but rather a public event, situated in a densely structured kinship system and underlined by the fact that burial was public, collective and ecclesiastical. The actual act of dying took place traditionally within the domestic sphere, in the company of kin folk and neighbours (Turner, 1987:127). Until as recently as the 1950s, Munley (1983:10) reports, people died at home surrounded by family, friends, children and the doctor who may have brought the person into the world.

The individual, Aries records (1991:9), was aware of impending death through warning signs handed down from generation to generation. Conscious that death was imminent, there was no expectation that death could be averted through medical therapies, and consequently there were no attempts to try (Martocchio, 1982:10). If the individual was not aware of his/her impending death, it was the responsibility of others to create this awareness (Aries, 1994:10). Consequently, death was acknowledged, not denied, with ritualistic processes to guide the individual and group in coping with its significance. Such a process, celebrated in the literature and pictorial representations of *Ars (Artes) Moriendi*, the art of dying, was a religious and spiritual endeavour, described by the fifteenth-century printer William Caxton as 'the craft for to deye for the helthe of mannes sowle' (Nuland, 1994:xvi).

The art of dying: a modern western way

Modern Western death is primarily institutionalised and impersonal largely taking place within the hospital setting (Manning, 1984:12).[1] Seen as a hygienic and often solitary death within the isolated space of a modern hospital contrasts greatly with the public but familial setting of the domestic situation of previous times (Turner, 1987:127).[2] Death-bed vigils became antiquated, and family participation was discouraged as dying people were ministered to by technical experts: death became a shameful and unacceptable event best dealt with in the sterile atmosphere of the hospital (Siebold, 1992:31). Twentieth century senses, according to Aries (1991:570), made more delicate by rapid advances in comfort, privacy, personal hygiene and ideas about asepsis, could no longer tolerate the sights and smells that, in pre-modern times, were accepted as part of daily living and dying. Sadly, modern death is driven by these dual motivations of concealing and sanitising (Nuland, 1994:xvi).

Modern western culture, in comparison to pre-modern times, is seen to be 'death denying' (Manning, 1984:12). According to Aries (1991:22-28), death is obliterated from our technological culture, which denies the reality of dying and, in so doing makes it difficult for the individual to imagine or understand it.[3] Concurring with this, Manning (1984:23) suggests that such death-denial stems from the fact that death embodies the unknown at the very deepest level, ultimately symbolising everything over which we can have no control. Indeed, Becker (1973) argues that such a denial is based on the 'fear that haunts the human animal like nothing else', the mainstream of human activity being to overcome this fear by denying, in some way, the final destiny. This fear of the unknown resonates throughout the literature on death and dying within our culture (Nuland, 1994:xv).

The secular, rationalistic, positivist notions of science are seen to figure largely in such a denial, for as Harrington explains, if 'fear of death is the mainstream of human conduct...the cure is obvious, abolish death...science is working on the problem' (cited in Becker, 1973:266). Whereas death was once a spiritual/religious event (Aries, 1991:13), there is now no longer the generalised metaphysical certainty of medieval times (Jung, 1955:204). In place of metaphysical speculation and an acceptance of death as destiny, modern medical discourse on dying privileges a cure oriented 'war' against death, driven by a technological imperative that sanctions the 'battle' at any cost.[4] The individual is no longer seen to die of 'natural causes'; instead, the notion of 'clinical death', which marginalises the idea of the inevitable normality of death is privileged: all death being avoidable, unnecessary or premature, and, but for the lack of medical attention is possible to avert[5] (Martocchio, 1982:25).

The side effect of such a technological revolution is that the individual increasingly faces the possibility of a lingering, isolated, and dehumanising dying in a bureaucratic medical setting (Munley, 1983:11). A communal orientation to dying has been replaced by the individualism of biomedical treatment; the sacred worldview has been displaced by science (ibid).

Nobody dies without being cured

The cure-oriented, scientific medicine of the biomedical model is the key determining factor in the present move to institutionalisation and dehumanisation of dying in our society. The President's Commission for the Study of Ethical Problems in Medicine (1982) identified the technological approach to medicine as 'perhaps the single most significant factor' in decision making about where and how dying takes place (cited in Ratcliff, 1989:264). Such cure-motivated care, with its emphasis on aggressive, eradicating therapies, is often not only inappropriate, but is also the core ingredient in the depersonalisation of death. Distressful therapies are offered long past their usefulness in a death-denying milieu, where symptom control and emotional care would have been much more appropriate (Blues and Zerwekh, 1984:3).[6] In the words of one observer, 'Nobody dies in this country without being cured' (Siebold, 1992:1). In such a cure-oriented system the physician has problems in acknowledging death, and ceasing treatment on the dying patient (Ratcliff, 1989 :264). Death is seen as a failure in a system where the training of the physician is based on his/her ability to cure (Siebold, 1992:19). In the words of Aries, 'death has ceased to be accepted as a natural, necessary phenomenon. Death is a failure, "a business lost". This is the attitude of the doctor, who claims the control of death as his mission in life' (1991:586).[7]

The dehumanisation of death

As outlined in the previous section on biomedicine, technologised care is also seen to have a vast potential for dehumanisation. The rational, reductionist approach has serious, negative implications in relation to the terminally ill, when, in the words of Munley,

> A dying person is treated as a thing, a machine, a guinea pig, a problem, an inferior, or an isolate without options in impersonal, sterile environments, one is robbed of human dignity, of the freedom to die in one's own way and in communion with one's fellows (1983:13).

The institutionalisation of dying has depersonalising aspects, not just from the technical treatment of the dying process, but also due to the disempowering nature of the socialrelations within the hospital setting. Control of information usually lies with the health professionals, which, coupled with the hierarchical relations which are the normal patterns within hospitals, makes the expression of individual autonomy and choice a real difficulty (Field and James, 1993:13). Unlike the *Ars Moreindi* of pre-modern times, the individual is often not aware of impending death, information is not given that the sick person is dying, ('closed awareness'), nor is reverence given to the solemn nature of the moment of death (Aries, 1994:11).

The research of Glaser and Strauss (1965) reveals that patients who died in hospital were abandoned by staff and left to struggle with complex feelings about their condition without much support. Indeed, the nearer to death, the less often their physicians visited them and the slower ancillary staff were to answer their calls. Sudnow's famous study (1967) gave innumerable examples of this dehumanising phenomenon which he titled 'social death', and refers to the time when the patient is still physiologically alive, but is treated socially and psychologically as if dead. Situational pressures and systemic forces of the hospital setting, where death is seen to be institutionalised to reduce its disruptive effect on the ongoing business of society, is seen as the motivating force behind such dehumanising behaviour (Siebold, 1992:33).

In such an institutional setting, not only is the individual denied choice and autonomy, but also feelings. Aries (1991:579) likens the present suppression of feelings in the name of denial of death to that of the sexual prudery of the last century. The feelings associated with dying and mourning, too intense for display, are given no chance of expression in a milieu designed for repression. As Aries explains,

> The denial of death is openly acknowledged as a significant trait of our culture. The tears of the bereaved have become comparable to the excretions of the diseased. Both are distasteful. Death has been banished...there is a conviction that the public demonstration of mourning, as well as its too-insistent or too-long private expression, is inherently morbid. Weeping is synonymous with hysteria. Mourning is a malady (1991:580).

Even in residential and nursing homes, where an increasing number of people now die, death is marginalised and seen primarily in terms of the practical problems which it creates for the staff. Most homes operate with a policy of 'closed awareness'; where all but the patient knows of the diagnosis and prognosis of their condition (Field and James, 1993:20). Disempowerment and depersonalisation are seen as the characteristics of the modern institutional nature of death.

Death has moved from the moral to the technical,[8] from the family to the hospital (Cassell, 1993:44). This confusion of the mechanical events of the death of the body with the personal and social nature of the passing of the person, according to Cassell (1993:46), confounds attempts to solve the essentially moral problems of the dying. Such an observation is backed up by the extensive literature on bioethics which seeks to interpret and reflect upon the moral dilemmas of dying created by scientific medicine: issues ranging from organ transplantation to the withdrawal of futile treatment. A concern with such issues is one of the rationales underpinning this present bioethical research.

One response to modern death: the hospice movement

The hospice movement arose out of the need to regain control over the normal life event of dying from physicians and institutions (Ratcliff, 1989:264; Rinaldi and Kearl, 1990). Reinscribing holistic care, a caring orientation, and a returning of control to the patient, hospice care moved awayfrom the technologised dying of the biomedical model to a philosophy that was inclusive of the physical, psychological, social and spiritual needs of the patient and their family (Manning, 1984). A grassroots reform movement, the hospice movement, the aim of which was to humanise terminal care, incorporated consumer desire for participation in health services, religious hopes for a return of the spiritual dimension, and a rebellion against authoritarian hospital systems (Siebold, 1992:28).

Central to the new discourse on death is the concept of '*death with dignity*', the *Ars Moriendi* of the twentieth century. A rhetoric developed against the excessive abuse of scientific biomedicine, the quality and not the quantity of life is seen as the principle value, underpinning such conceptualisations as the 'Dying Patient's Bill of Rights', and living wills (Martocchio, 1982:27).

Exploring a different 'way': KHS's discourse on dying

The discourse of KHS privileges the opportunity to return dying to the domestic sphere, surrounded by family, friends and neighbours, if that is the individual's choice. A spiritual, Buddhist based discourse which is concerned with the holistic needs of the individual patient and their family it marginalises the secular, reductionist, dehumanising aspects of the biomedical approach to death, characteristic of our modern Western society. Emphasising the importance of choice for the individual, in how and where they wish to die, the KHS discourse seeks to reinscribe power to the dying patient, where it has been marginalised by our present day practices in caring for the dying.

A twenty four hour service, which incorporates the contribution of dedicated volunteers, KHS offers holistic follow-up, which includes not only the patient but also the family. Such follow-up starts at the time of referral through to bereavement counselling of the families. This holistic orientation includes the psycho-social-physical-spiritual needs of the patient and their family.

Although the KHS discourse reinscribes the primacy of non-judgemental, compassionate care, over a technical/mechanistic notion of care, it does not marginalise a respect for the clinical skills of pain management and symptom relief of bio-medicine. In short, KHS's discourse can be seen to be in a creative relationship with mainstream biomedicine, not just a simple opposition to, or rejection of, reductionist biomedical ideas.

It is *this creative relationship between the emergent discourse of KHS and biomedicine that will be THE central focus directing the ongoing interpretation of data.* The continuing theme of such an analysis of KHS's discourse will be that it can be viewed as a *deconstructive reading of mainstream ideas.* Such a view would see KHS's 'talk' about death and dying actively constructed in relation to ideas considered problematic in biomedicine. From such a perspective, the KHS discourse would be seen to be developed from a reading of biomedicine, but one which in effect, seeks to hear, to say, and thus to act upon important and constructive notions (as perceived by KHS) which are marginalised or silenced in biomedicine. Equally, KHS's discourse can be seen to be actively seeking to silence or suppress biomedical notions that members of this organisation believe to be counterproductive or damaging in their work with the terminally ill. KHS's discourse can thus be perceived as a reading of the hegemonic medicalised and technologised notions of dying: a reading with a strong investment in creating an alternative reality in working with the dying.

The focus and context of the 'talk' of KHS can be seen to be in a direct relationship with biomedicine: a focus which will remain at the heart of the interpretation developed. It is important, however, to note two caveats to such an interpretation. Firstly, it is my (rather than KHS's) interpretation that Karuna's alternative discourse on dying operates on a 'deconstructed centre' of biomedicine.[9] Such an interpretation has been constructed through the insights of postmodern writers on deconstruction (as outlined in Chapter 2). There is *no* expectation that members of KHS have any consciously articulated awareness that either they, or the discourse they are immersed in, can be viewed as 'reading' biomedicine (actively silencing notions deemed central with aview to privileging and constructing an alternative reading).[10] In short, notions of silencing and privileging are postmodern notions, not ideas which emerged from the participants interviewed.

Nevertheless, this does not negate that *members of KHS were very conscious of, and expressed clearly in interviews, the notion that they wished to develop a service very different from biomedicine.* It was the articulation of this concern to create a service different to mainstream health practices, as well as participants description of KHS's difference *via negitiva* to biomedicine (as will be discussed in the following chapter), which formed the basis of the rationale for the interpretation which was developed. Participants defined what they say about KHS's difference in terms directly related to the hegemonic discourse of biomedicine. The participants directly articulated the connection between these two discourses. In short, to both the participants and myself, the relationship between KHS and biomedicine *is significant.* Although I initiated the process of translating such a connection into terms arising from the work of writers on deconstruction, such an interpretation can be seen as referring to a process that is actually recorded as happening. Consequently, the second caveat to this interpretation is that, although the notions associated with deconstruction which are used at the interface between biomedicine and KHS's emergent discourse are owned as my own construct, these ideas can be applied to a clearly articulated and stated process owned by the members of this organisation. Participants may not have conceptually thought in terms of silencing and privileging (or deconstructing or reading biomedicine), but through their 'talk' they actively sought to describe who they are and who they are not in relation to biomedicine (ideas which will be further developed in the following chapter).

Conclusion

The discussion so far has emphasised that KHS's primary concern focuses on incorporating holistic ways of talking about death and dying. By emphasising the psycho-social-spiritual needs of the terminally ill, KHS's 'talk' has been situated in the hospice response to dying which seeks to suppress the destructive, depersonalising, dehumanising aspects of modern technologised death.

At the same time as resisting the dehumanising influence of medicalisation, KHS creates a respectful space for the clinical skills and knowledge that assist in the holistic, comfort orientated care of the patient, (i.e. symptom relief and pain management). This complex and creative relationship to biomedicine (introduced in this chapter) will remain the central focus of the ongoing interpretation developed.

Notes

1 According to Manning, (1984:12) at the turn of the century, 80% of all deaths on average occurred at home; by 1976 the figure had dropped to 20%. By the mid-1960s, 66% of all deaths in the UK occurred in hospitals or other places caring for the sick, and by 1989 this had risen to 71% with only 23% of 'home deaths' (Field and James, 1993:12). Rinaldi and Kearl (1990:284) provide an estimate that 80% of people now die in institutions when they write, 'With the profanation of death, the idea of death became a matter of pornography, and its incidence institutionally hidden. Where in the early 1900s only 10 to 20 % of people died outside their homes, today over 80 % die in institutions.'

2 Kellehear's recent research (1990:12) contextualises this trend toward institutional death to the Australian setting. Updating Fulton's findings

(1972) that the bulk of dying occurs in hospitals and/or nursing home institutions, Kellehear uses Australian reseach (Malden et al., 1984; Howe, 1982) to point out that 'Australia is no exception to this trend' (1990:12). For example, Australian statistics by Malden and associates (1984) indicated that from follow up recorded deaths of patients from the Royal Prince Alfred Hospital, Sydney, and the Royal North Shore Hospital, Sydney, 73% of those patients died in hospital, 9% died in terminal care (TNC) institutions, and the remainder at home. Hunt's research comparing such institutionalised death with the experience of dying at home suggests a poignant and significant difference. Of the research on hospital deaths, Hunt writes (1992:1297) 'the majority of studies of dying in hospitals present negative and dismal pictures of the process', whilst on home deaths, 'in contrast to this, there is an increase in accounts by terminally ill writers of their attempts to live the final stages of their lives at home in productive and satisfying ways' (ibid).

3 As will be elaborated on in later chapters such a denial of meaning is also reflected in the present rationalistic ethical approach to issues of death and dying. As Barnard (1988:395) states, 'Human beings are creatures who seek love and meaning in the face of death. The impact of this dimension of human existence is rarely attended to in discussions of medical ethics, where it is overshadowed by the justification and application of principles and efforts to balance competing rights and obligations in particular situations.'

4 Corbett and Hai (1979:38) describe modern death as the individual 'surrounded with and enslaved by their own unbridled technology. Transplants, haemodialysis, intravenous therapy, nasogastric feeding, complete respiratory support - there is always something else to be done'.

5 Scott (1987:343) situates this phenomenon historically when he writes that 'death also changed with the birth of modern medical knowledge. Whereas death had been the end of a disease, a completion that was signified by the mere disposal of dead bodies, with the emergence of pathological anatomy, focussed on the corpse, death became a process for discovery...It seemed to promise the possibility for open, lucid mastery, for hope to establish a remarkable control by knowledge over the deteriorating body.'

6 Kohut and Kohut (1984:24) partly attributed this overtreatment to the self-blame of doctors and nurses when 'catastrophic disease is not halted. With a tremendous arsenal of weapons available in fighting the disease, physicians are prone to prescribe transfusions, medications and ambulation when in retrospect the most humane prescription or action is discharge from the hospital and sending the patient home.'

7 Holman (1990:17-18) when pointing out the 'unspoken yet pervasive attitude that death represents failure of medical expertise' suggests that 'given the highly technological and scientific society we live in, death can represent both existential and individual, personal failure. When health professionals assume the responsibility of defying death, they must, to some degree, perhaps unconsciously, deny their personal feelings; they sacrifice the human needs and dignity of their clients in the process.'

8 Technical innovations even impacted on the definition given to the meaning of death. The Ad Hoc Committee of the Harvard Medical School (1968), moved the definition of death from 'heart death' to 'brain death' criteria because of increasing need for transplantable organs (Bayertz, 1992:410).

9 The term 'deconstructed centre' has been coined to suggest that the ideas being referred to here are not marginal to biomedicine. The assumption is that the ideas that concern members of KHS are at the very 'centre' of biomedicine. Consequently, the alternative discourse of KHS can be seen to be touching the core of biomedical ways of seeing.

10 Or as Norris (1987:19) has decribed the deconstructive process 'dismantling of conceptual oppositions, the taking apart of hierarchical systems of thought which can then be reinscribed within a different order of textual signification.'

8 Silencing the 'technological imperative'

> The very identity of a scientific discourse is revealed only at the site of its competition with others (Rawlinson, 1987:375).

Throughout the language/texts, KHS's difference has been defined, *via negativa,* not only by statements of distinction, i.e. 'what KHS is', but also by statements of contrast, i.e. 'what it is not'. Invariably, *such statements of contrast referred to the bio-medical model,* as seen by the following language/texts,

> The medical model doesn't really sit very comfortably with the spiritual (EQ).

> (On an)...oncology ward, (I have) seen a lot of things happen I have not really liked. People not given facts. hospitals are intimidating places, even the most assertive person is disempowered. (There are) real power structures which effects patients and their family and disempowers staff as well. So you see things happen that you really don't think are right but you really don't think that you have the power to change (EQ).

> I believe nurses may care in the hospital they often don't have the time to care (EQ).

> (In a) hospital someone else takes over. Because of shifts, you are more cut off...institution, role more circumscribed (EQ).

An assumption underpinning this work is that the notions incorporated in any discourse create meaning by privileging one set of ideas at the cost of suppressing the conceptual opposite. As outlined in Chapter 2, the insights provided by writers who use deconstruction are used to provide ways of looking at or exposing the notions which are silenced by this very act of constructing meaning through language. With such an understanding, it becomes as important to look, not only at what is being said or expressed in a discourse, but also at what is being suppressed. The notions expressed in KHS's spiritual discourse create meaning, not only by ideas stated or emphasised, but just as importantly by what is avoided in the 'talk'.

As has been shown by the statements in the introduction to this chapter, members of KHS clearly express in their holistic, spiritual 'talk' a desire to articulate ideas which will silence notions central to the biomedical approach (hierarchial institutional power and physiological reductionism) to caring for the dying. Consequently, in exploring with a deconstructive lens what is actually said about KHS's difference, one possibility is to see in this discourse the active suppression of notions to do with the practice of reductionist, hierarchial biomedicine.

When reading a text, writers on deconstruction are not just concerned with isolating notions hidden in a discourse, but are also, just as importantly, concerned with how meaning can be constructed by giving voice to ideas not being said.[1] The task is to replace the meaning created by exclusion and repression by allowing the expression of alternative 'reading'; or another way of seeing the ideas expressed in the text. By taking participants statements about KHS's difference as examples of discourse, the proposition is that it is possible to see, through interpreting how meaning is constructed in these texts, that the 'talk' of KHS is, in many ways, acting to express or privilege holistic, spiritual ideas which are marginalised or deleted from the biomedical approach to dying. The KHS discourse on the care for the terminally ill can thus be understood to be not only silencing important notions central to the biomedical approach, but simultaneously, actively and creatively articulating alternative ideas, or ways of seeing, which are stifled by a reductionist physiological approach to death.

The proposition born of such an understanding is that, by exploring the connection between biomedicine and KHS's spiritual discourse, the meaning making and construction of reality of both discourses becomes clearer. As Ralinson's statement (1987:375) in the beginning of this chapter suggests, it is only at the site of competition with other discourses that the identity of any discourse is revealed.[2]

An exploration of how meaning is created in KHS's discourse of difference is consequently set in the context of the literature and research on the bio-medical model. As this model (biomedicine) is predicated on notions of scientific positivism, the initial discussion will be an exploration of modernist ideas of scientific rationalism. The holistic, spiritual discursive practices of KHS, it is argued, marginalise such a construction of reality. The inclusion of a spiritual dimension to the individual and family, *ipso facto,* silences the familiar reductionist, physiological, subjectivity of the biomedical discourse.

The scientific discourse

In contrast to the elusive dimension of the spiritual discourse, the modernist scientific beliefs which underpin our medical interventions are based on positivist, scientific notions of *neutrality* and *objectivity*, conceptualised through a linear, teleological rationality (Lather, 1991:105).[3] Indeed, according to Cassell (1991a:x), the dominance of science has led to the widely held and crippling prejudice that no knowledge is real unless it is scientific-objective and measurable (empirical). The discourse of KHS, by way of contrast, whilst respectful of the knowledge base of biomedicine, recognises the possibility of other ways of knowing, incorporating an epistemology inclusive of a spiritual metaphysic.

The philosophical foundation of the scientific concern with the body was inscribed by Descartes's philosophical grand theory of the division of the person into mind (*res cogitans*) and body (*res extensa*) (Foss, 1989:166; Freund and McGuire, 1991:226; Kleinman, 1986). Such a philosophy, known as Cartesian dualism, was, according to Foucault (1973), practically translated into clinical and pathological anatomy by what he describes as the 'clinical gaze': an emphasis on direct clinical observation and physical examination. The body became disassociated from the person, an object for study and intervention. Foucault (1973) argues that 'scientific' knowledge developed through the 'clinical gaze' gave physicians enormous social prestige and influence, not only in defining reality but also in identifying deviance and social disorder (Turner, 1987:11).

Underpinned by notions of rationalism and a belief in progress through science, this reductionist, physiological orientation directs an engineering approach to medicine (Plowles, 1973). Such an approach is informed by an *unquestioned* acceptance of notions such as knowledge, progress, truth, and rationality (Fox, 1991:722). In our technologised society, Comaroff argues (1982:59), science is 'depoliticised': the latent meanings implicit in bio-medicine carry the very assertion that it is free from the influence of symbol and value.[4]

Scientific values however, although reified as objectivity and truth, are more concerned with *mastery and control* (Ratcliff, 1989:174). The metaphors used by the founding fathers, during the time of the conceptualisation of Western science, provide invaluable insights into the historical construction of the underlying value base of the scientific enterprise. Rather than claims to holistic, interconnectedness, the men of the Scientific Revolution used strong words of force and mastery to express the ideology motivating their work. Bacon wished to 'have the power to conquer and subdue her (nature), to shake her to her foundations' (cited in Ratcliff, 1989:174), as he believed that 'you have but to follow and as it were, hound nature in her wanderings, and you will be able, when you like, to lead and drive her afterwards to the same place again' (cited in Jecker, 1991:6).[5] Descartes similarly hoped that the new science meant that human beings would be the 'masters' and 'possessors' of nature (ibid). This metaphor of control has become a powerful determinant in both lay and professional thinking (Comaroff, 1982:56). Western medicine, not surprisingly, is considered a most invasive enterprise, as such values encourage invasive technological solutions to problems (Ratcliff, 1989:172).

In view of this historical background, it is argued, when the myth of neutrality of positivist science is deconstructed, one important concern underlying the rhetoric of objectivity appears to be control.[6] This notion of control, silenced in the discursive practices of KHS, is privileged and central to the scientific discourse underpinning biomedicine.

Similarly, science also privileges *rationalism.*[7] This scientific rational calculability, which is a given within our social structure and discourses, is not necessarily an uncontested fact of existence, but arguably, the result of an historical development of the dialectical process between the emergent philosophies of science and the secular.[8]

Such scientific rationalism impacts not only on the constructed subjectivity of the patient, but also on issues of reverence for the human body. The explanation of the body through empirical evidence which silences 'nonnatural' metaphysics, according to Weber (1958:139), sanctions a 'disenchantment' of the world, where phenomena once held in awe or reverence are stripped of their special qualities and become ordinary. The reified notion of the human body, through this ideology of rationalism, becomes one of a disenchanted entity requiring no special reverence, as opposed to the previously held notion of a spiritual temple worthy of respect (Freund and McGuire, 1991:225). Such a discourse marginalises not only the holistic spiritual significance of the individual identity, but also the sanctity and reverence of their body parts. Such a rational reductionist discourse is most obviously evidenced in the language of the organ transplantation trade (Shaw et al., 1991; Teo, 1991).

This modernist belief in rationality is now challenged as but one discourse in the construction of reality. Insight, existential meaning, and the possibility of a transcendent reality are all ideas privileged within the KHS discourse which would marginalise such a secular, rational discourse.

The ideology underpinning the scientific enterprise is an optimism which sees human salvation as being achieved through technology, with particular emphasis on the illusion of *medical salvation* (Borges, 1986:26). According to Smith (1992:117), only a century ago there was a shared awareness of the limitations of medical intervention, but today, the perceived power of the scientific technological medicine is enormous: high expectations for 'medical miracles' abound (Gillis et al., 1989:12). Unfortunately, the enthusiasm for the latest scientific breakthroughs, inherent in the salvation ideology, has led to exaggerated expectations and uncritical acceptance of medical innovation (Dutton, 1988:4). The force within biomedicine driving such exaggerated expectations has been titled the 'technological imperative'.

The technological imperative

> It (hospital) is more kind of boom, boom, you have to do this (EQ).

Back in 1968, Fuchs coined the term the 'technological imperative' to name that process within the medical tradition which gave primacy to interventions based on doing whatever was technically possible (Fuch, 1968:192). A technological optimism, based on high hopes of achievement, a curative orientation, an underestimation of risks, a suppression of doubts and an assumption of unlimited resources (Dutton, 1988:351-2) provided the rhetoric and ideology driving this new *raison d'etre* for medical intervention. The overriding ethic in clinical decision making became that of doing what was technically possible: doing everything possible, even if there is a very low probability of benefiting the patient (Jonsen, 1990:51; Short, 1985).[9] The medical technology, once implemented, is seen to quickly beget more technology.[10] In such a milieu, diagnosis, not treatment, becomes a culture, creating excessive use of technological intervention[11] which does not necessarily add to the possibility of cure.[12] Such a diagnostic culture seeks to label, even when it is obviously unable to treat (Wolf and Berle, 1981:17-21). This approach is predicated on the scientific method, with modern technology as the tools of trade (Wanzer et al., 1984). Such an interpretation of medical need, in the face of increasing technical innovation, is inherently elastic and open-ended, providing neither a reliable guide for patient benefit nor a firm foundation for doctor obligation (Goodman, 1991:179).[13]

Such technology[14] is applied extensively throughout our society, from the extremely young and fragile, to the hopelessly ill and irretrievably old (Melski, 1992:1517), creating alarm, concern and debate about escalating costs for expensive interventions which consume an increasing proportion of the public finances (Aaron and Schwartz, 1985; Brody, 1987; Ellard, 1991; Menzel, 1990; Morreim, 1985). The decision to use such technology is compelled by pressures which favour the continuing of treatment at all costs. Such pressures include an inability to accept the inevitability of death, the desire to provide the patient with 'every chance', fear of judgment error and litigation, and the fear of the burden of personal guilt, created from not having tried everything possible for the patient (Dunstan and Shinebourne, 1989:178). This vicious cycle of commitment, where the patient is invaded by the arsenal of technological possibilities in a medical milieu of unrealistic hope, denial of death, and technological rationalism, is the very essence of the 'technological imperative'. Intervention decisions are driven by the state of the art, not by considered concern about the patient's emotional, physical, and spiritual experience[15] (Fuchs, 1968:192).

Such a positivist, problem-solving orientation to specialised medicine (Turner, 1990:4) has developed in response to the scientific epistemological assumptions, popularly known as the bio-medical model.

The bio-medical model

> Contemporary biomedicine has been criticised for its reductionism and dualism, the objectification of the patient, and isolation from his or her social and cultural environment. The reliance on technology and the quest for objective - that is,scientific - measures of disease through the

development of complex diagnostic technology has led to an obliteration of the patient as a whole being removed from his suffering and to the reduction of the human being to a mechanical body (Finkler, 1991:77).

Biomedicine is based on a number of assumptions about the body, disease and ways of knowing, principal notions being the mind-body dualism, physical reductionism, specific aetiology, 'machine' metaphor, and orientation to regimen and control (Freund and McGuire, 1991:226-228; Turner, 1987; Zaner, 1990).

This model sees medicine to be guided by objective facts, unaffected by the wider social, cultural and political forces. A biological rather than social focus dominates the paradigm, with the 'doctrine of specific aetiology' placing disease as a separate entity to be explored within the body of the individual (Mishler, 1981:16). A mechanistic model of health, where the body is seen as a machine, affected by its chemistry as well as its physics, adopts the Cartesian duality of mind and body, seeing medicine as only concerned with repairing that physiological machine (Jacob, 1988:32-5; Finkler, 1991:1). Medical scientists view disease as an explicit ontological entity, the 'conquest' of which takes place by aggressive interventions into the body of the individual (Jecker, 1991:6). The aggressive and invasive nature of the present biomedical model is a result, not only of its historical situation in the scientific discourse of control, but, as importantly, in its origination from the medical belief system dubbed *allopathy,* characterised by 'heroic' and invasive treatments such as bloodletting, purging, blistering, vomiting and mediating with powerful drugs and poisons (Freund and McGuire, 1991:220). During the formative stages of biomedicine, *allopathy* became the hegemonic discourse over the less dangerous alternatives of competing approaches such as homoeopathy (ibid).

This reductionist orientation toward the individual is revealed in the depersonalisation of the language of biomedicine, which emphasises the disease or organ but not the patient (Anspach, 1990). A reification of the body as an object, separate from the person who inhabits it, denies the social meanings embodied in symptoms, diagnoses, therapy, and even in the very experience of illness itself (Freund and McGurie, 1991:217). This reified reality of the objectified 'disease-thing' is often treated as more real than the person's feelings (ibid). In short, the doctor is seen to 'treat diseases rather than patients' (Anspach, 1990). In the words of one participant,

> People loose part of that personhood when they go into hospital...it is not your space...it very much belongs to the people whose rules you don't understand, you are never quite sure if you are complying with the rules or not (EQ).

This separation of the disease that underlies the suffering from both the person and the suffering itself, as though the scientific entity of disease is more real and more important than the person and the suffering, according to Cassell (1991a:ix), is the central paradox of biomedicine. This is backed up by Freund and McGuire (1991:151), who suggest that health professionals working within the biomedical discourse cause more suffering by (silencing) failing to acknowledge or deal with the personal meanings the patient attaches to illness.

This reduction of the person to an object of study, a physiological 'thing' to be 'worked on', is a recurring theme expressed by those who write or speak about their experiences with biomedicine. Courtenay (1993), when describing the tragic story of his haemophiliac son's death through blood product contracted AIDS, articulates with dramatic clarity the psychological distress caused by the reductionist 'gaze' of the hospital physician. Courtenay's literary expression of two exaggerated physician related incidences which occured during his son's short life (one as a baby and one near death) will be related here as a way of more fully describing the intellectual concepts presently being discussed. The intent in providing such examples is to demonstrate by example the inherent danger in the biomedical lens. The suggestion is not that health professionals invariably do, or must always act with such callous indifference, but rather that the reductionist biomedical discourse normalises such 'talk'. Courtenay also acknowledges in his book a gratitude for the physicians who treated his son with compassion and understanding.

The first such incident involves the reaction of the hospital physician to his baby son's haemophiliac induced head bleed. Courtenay brings this incident to life when he writes (1993:54) of the hospital physican's verbal reaction to discovering the baby's condition as,

> Extraordinary! Gentlemen, you will spend your entire medical careers and never see anything like this again. Mr..er, the photographer here, will record it for a case study I intend to write. What's the umbrella for? I see..lighting, bounces light back into the subject. Ah-ha, I see, a reflector, a photographer's reflector. Will you use flash? We want all the details. You must shoot every angle, we may never get another chance. See how perfect, gentlemen. See here, you can poke your finger into the cranium. It's all blood, a massive, quite outstanding haematoma. Here, come on gentlemen, touch it. What do you think is the cause? Anyone like to hazard a guess?

A similar incident during the time of his son's dying reinforced for Courtenay the notion that for the whole of his son's life and illness (haemophilia starts at birth) the biomedical approach to Damon (his son) was to see him as 'a thing, a curiosity' (1993:654). This time the incident was set of by a case of *Herpes Zoster*. Courtenay writes (1993:644),

> At first the medico seemed pleasant enough. That was until he saw Damon's shingles. He brought his hands up to his chest and smiled broadly, unable to contain his delight. 'God! I've never seen anything as good as this! There must be two hundred blisters!' He rose quickly and crossed to a desk and searched through a drawer for a magnifying glass, returning to the examination couch with it. 'On the legs and feet, under the sole, that's *very* unusual.' He looked up and placed the glass down on the couch and

clapped his hands in delight, thrilled at what he had seen.

Such objectification is not reserved only for the extraordinary but is part of the everyday experience of the biomedical approach, prompting those with a long term experience with illness to call for a more humanising approach. Walsh (1992:6), facing his own death through cancer and having endured the ravages of extensive chemotherapy, argues that 'there needs to be a greater emphasis put on the patient as a person, not a number or a disease'. Furthermore, Galloway (1992), a teenage girl who has spent a life time in and out of hospitals fighting a crippling and disfiguring disease, makes the plea that health professionals understand that 'patients are not a collection of bladders, bowels and various body parts. They are real people with real emotions and real feelings.'

Central to understanding illness and affliction, Cassell argues, is the individual's search for meaning and an essential coherence to their world (Cassell, 1991a). These ideas are paradoxically marginalised by the biomedical model. One participant expressed the issue as follows,

> The medical model doesn't really sit very comfortably with the spiritual...and that is something that is actually changing slowly and surely, and there are more people becoming more aware (EQ).

It must be stressed that the notion under discussion is the inherent danger in biomedical discourse not the personal qualities of the health professional who are daily players in this discourse. Empathy and compassion are qualities that health professionals both value and bring to their interaction with patients (Bailey, 1996; Baillie, 1996; Bennett, 1995; Cassell, 1991; Jecker, 1991b; Jonsen, 1990; Kearsley, 1993; La Monica et al., 1987; Morse et al., 1992; Pellegrino, 1979). As will be discussed in later chapters, it is the discourse rather than the indivual which predominantly determines the expression (or repression) of such qualities. The one individual, it will be shown, can and will act very differently in settings defined by dissimilar discourses.[16]

The KHS discourse, far from marginalising notions of meaning, actually acknowledges such notions through its holistic, and spiritual orientation to care. There is also within the Karuna discourse, a stated awareness of the negative implications of the reductionist stance of biomedicine,

> The medical model treats the disease and the rest of the person can look after itself (EQ).

> ...hospital ward where you may die in the middle of the night alone and in pain and terrified (EQ).

If contextualised to the already outlined discussion of KHS's discourse on the patient, it can be seen that the caring, compassionate, supportive, holistic 'talk' of this service incorporates a much richer notion of what it is to be a patient. Such holistic ideas stand as a deconstructed centre[17] of the biomedical social construction of the patient.

As has been pointed out previously, although KHS privileges this much richer subjectivity of the individual patient, it does not completely marginalise biomedicine's contribution, especially in the area of respect for clinical skills[18] and physician competence. The discursive practices of KHS, whilst marginalising much of the reductionist patient subjectivity of biomedicine, privilege such skills in the area of pain management and symptom control.

The 'for profit' motive

An engineering approach to medicine, where health professionals are perceived as biotechnicians, has led to the development of an industry, shaped by profit and the income orientations of its key participants (Ratcliff, 1989:173).

Labelled as the 'medical-industrial complex' (Relman, 1980 :963), such a health care infrastructure is seen to create problems with overuse and fragmentation of services, with an overemphasis on technology (ibid). Indeed, medicine and commercial interests are seen as a powerful partnership, creating real problems in interpretation of need and service delivery (Rowland, 1992:12). Technological innovations are favoured, with quality of care being defined in terms of whatis technologically possible (Ratcliff, 1989:182). Such a tendency of the profit-making sector to emphasise procedures and technology is seen to operate on a notion of *cure*[19] to the exclusion of personal *care.*[20] Such personal care, whether provided by physicians, nurses, or other health-care practitioners, is considered expensive and less likely to produce large profits than the item-by-item application of technology.[21]

As seen by the following statements, the discursive practices of KHS silence the profit motive central to the biomedical model,

> Karuna (is a) spiritually based organisation, that it is not based on profit or that it is run on more pure motivation, and that it does have a spiritual basis (EQ).
>
> If they are just there to do a job and a paid job and they haven't got that commitment and they haven't got that motivation, then that is not going to translate...they are the things that you can't quantify with dollars (EQ).

Medicocentric power

Historically, the marriage of science and medicine was instituted within the context of support by the financial interests of affluent, bourgeoisie foundations. The Flexner Report of 1910, through the backing of the Carnegie and Rockefeller Foundation, selected, funded, and legitimised the prototype medical schools along the lines of the John Hopkins Medical School (Turner, 1990:8). Through such a social and political phenomenon, the biomedical model then became tied by class, race and gender to powerful men in foundations and government. The state-supported monopoly to practise medicine became, without competition, professionally dominated by the physician (Fisher, 1991:179). Within just a few decades, such professional dominance was virtually total through state-legitimated control which eliminated, coopted, or subordinated all competing health professionals (Freund and McGuire, 1991:219). The 'fact' that disease/illness is located within the body has always ensured medical dominance in biomedicine, because only physicians possess the knowledge and skills to identify the problem, and the patient must thus remain epistemologically and socially subservient (Armstrong, 1987:1214). Central to the Foucaultian notion of the subjectivity of patienthood is the disempowerment exercised through expert control, through knowledge/power of the body (Fox, 1993:29). Because few people in modern society possess advanced medical knowledge or technical skills, the ability to control such knowledge is the basis of rewards, power and privilege, which limits the access of others (Freud and McGuire, 1991). The power and control of such medicocentrism is an important characteristic of biomedicine.

Such medicocentric power is acknowledged and negatively perceived within the language/texts, as seen by the following,

> In the average ward the doctor comes in and makes the decisions, the nurse implements, the senior pharmacist implements and so on, it is very hierarchical (EQ).

> Nurses are inclined to be a bit bossy anyway and the medical profession is inclined to be in control (EQ).

Such control is not just restricted to the power relations within a health institution, but is increasingly seen to be invading all aspects of human life. Such a process of social control has been termed the 'medicalizing of society' (Zola, 1990:401). Understandably, the area of death and dying is one such dimension of human existence in which biomedicine has played a formative role.

KHS's holistic discourse suppresses such notions of medico-centric power and control. The KHS response to the dying is built on a democratic multidisciplinary approach to empowering the individual patient and their family. As previously detailed, KHS was not the extension of a medical institution but instigated in the community by a Buddhist monk who is a physiotherapist. Although the staff of KHS are highly respectful of the valuable input of medical specialist and general practitioners, at present this organisation does not employ a physician. The discourses central to KHS's construction of meaning (Hospice/palliative care; Buddhist; Spiritual and Death and Dying) all include a holisitic respect for the autonomous wishes of the client, as well as a vision of democratic organisational relationships.

Conclusion

> Karuna can go on and do a lot of good if it stays half an inch above the medical model...if we had six Karunas treating people in their homes so they don't have to die in some cold white ward (EQ).

The underlying theme of this discussion has been the way in which meaning is constructed in KHS's holistic, spiritual discourse in relation to notions underpinning biomedicine. To achieve this end, an outline has been sketched of the reductionist, mechanistic, positivist, rational, secular, scientific discourse known as the biomedical model. Such a one dimensional discourse stands in stark contrast to the preceding discussions on spirituality, Buddhism and palliative care/hospice.

By using the insights of writers who engage in deconstructing texts, it has been proposed that both KHS's discourse and that of biomedicine can be best understood at the point where they meet. The 'talk' of KHS has been shown to be in a direct relationship to that of biomedicine: actively silencing, privileging and constructing alternative ways of seeing, to the reductionist physiological perspective on dying.

The biomedical model, it is argued, not only marginalises, but actively excludes core ingredients of spirituality and holism, as seen by this concluding summary by Hewa and Hetherington,

> Everything that happens to a patient can be explained in scientific terms. Psychology, spirituality and emotions are not regarded as important aspects of medicine, nor are they part of medical jargon. Therefore, aspects of the patient's problems which are accessible to scientific intervention and analysis will take priority, while those aspects which are less well comprehended (emotions, spirituality, social well-being) are likely to be ignored. This results in doing what is technologically possible, rather than in doing what may be in the best interests of the patient, all things considered (1990:181).

Notes

1 Lemert would refer to this process as replacing the deconstructed centre by the freeplay of discursive expression (1992:31).

2 An ongoing theme of this work has been that KHS to a large degree defines itself in relation to its dissimilarity to biomedicine. Consequently, the conviction is that it is at the interface between these discourses that insights can be gained both about KHS and biomedicine. The intersection between biomedicine and KHS's emerging discourse has been chosen and will remain the central focus for this work. In exploring this connection through a deconstructive process, the following conceptual binary opposites (expressed as deconstruction graphics) will be articulated - holism /reductionism; spirituality/secularism; democratic

organisation/hierarchical structure; patient choice /medicocentrism; significance of death/denial of death; person/disease; values/objectivity; empowerment/control; commitment/employment; support/criticism; and comprehensive care/technical intervention. By comparison the KHS discourse of genesis was seen to be absorbing, rather than competing with hospice discourse. It thus sufficed to situate KHS's discourse within the context of hospice/palliative care rather than explore the meaning making connection.

3 As Harding explains (1986:245) 'All versions of the scientific world view take science to be a totalising theory; it has been assumed that anything and everything worth understanding can be explained or interpreted within the assumptions of modern science.'

4 Harding (1986:245) talks about the alternative to rational science when she writes, 'yet there is another world hidden from the consciousness of science - the world of emotions, feelings, political values; of the individual and collective unconscious; of social and historical particularity explored by novels, drama, poetry, music, and art - within which we all live most of our waking and dreaming hours under constant threat of its increasing infusion by scientific rationality.'

5 Bird (1976:45) refers to this as the 'Baconian Dream' which was to 'extend the power and domination of the human race itself over the universe.'

6 According to Fay, by marking out the 'world' as a world of observable phenomena, subject to general laws, it is constructing reality from the viewpoint of how control can be gained over such a 'world' (1975:40).

7 Indeed, the modernist notion of the certainty, the superiority and self-confidence promised by the 'progressive' values of rationality is seen as the hallmark of modern Western society (Bauman, 1988:220).

8 Berger and Luckman (1966) views such rationalism as a human product, externalised and objectified; a reified world to be experienced as a strange facticity over which there is no human control.

9 Pellegrino writes extensively on the dangers of such a force in medicine. When discussing issues associated with human value and purpose, he writes, 'the sciences are too susceptible to seductions of the "technological imperative" to be safe guides through such intricacies' (1979:4).

10 Willis (1994:18) describes this phenomenon as 'technological determinism'. Such technology, he suggests, through the necessary division of labour needed to implement it, creates the hierarchy which today constitutes the social structure of health care delivery characterised by medical dominance (ibid).

11 Cassell (1993:32) equates medicine's rampant use of technology with the broom in 'The Sorcerer's Apprentice'. He delineates four factors which physicians need to confront to bring the dangers of such excessive use of technology into check. These factors include doctors learning to tolerate ambiguity, resist the lure of the immediate, cease fearing uncertainty and rechannel their response to wonder.

12 Palmer and Short (1989:173) record that 'medical technology has been

subjected to much criticism because of the perception in some quarters that, at worst, it may do more harm than good, and that in many instances efficacy has not been demonstrated prior to its adoption.. An impressive array of evidence, reported mainly in the medical literature and often based on the work of doctors, has raised questions about a wide range of individual technological developments, including antenatal foetal heart rate monitoring, intensive care and coronary care units, computerised axial tomography (CAT), magnetic resonance imaging (MRI), chemotherapy for cancer, and many of the more complex surgical procedures.'

13 Jennett (1986:127) writes of the hidden aspects of assessing such patient benefit in relation to cancer treatments in such a cure oriented technogical system when he writes about the burden of long term side effect, and the psychological disturbance caused by the mutilating effect of such treatments. He concludes that 'Doctors also often underestimate the cost to patients of compliance with continuing treatment - not only in patients themselves but in other family members.'

14 For the purpose of this research, definition of medical technology will be taken to be 'the drugs, devices and medical and surgical procedures used in medical care and the organisational and supportive systems within which such care is provided' (Calnan and Williams, 1992:236).

15 According to Jennett (1994:862) 'doctors are even sometimes accused of being wedded to technology for its own sake, rather than for the patient's benefit, particularly when the result is to prolong life that is of questionable quality. Technology is also often seen as distancing doctors from their patients, consequently replacing or reducing the touching and talking that used to be at the centre of the doctor-patient encounter. In this respect technology is sometimes suspected of having a dehumanising effect on medical practice.'

16 Writers such as Barnard (1988:403) express serious doubts about whether the biomedical model could incorporate support and holistic care as seen by his statement that 'it is open to question whether the modern hospital, and the fragmentation of medical care among the myriad specialties (including a host of professions competing for the role of caring for the 'whole person'), can provide such a holding environment.'

17 This notion of a 'deconstructed centre' has been introduced and elaborated on both in chapter 2 and earlier in this chapter. In this context this term refers to the idea that KHS's spiritual discourse on holism, gives voice to and articulates *central* or *cardinal* (rather than marginal) notions which are suppressed in biomedicine. In so doing, the 'talk' of KHS does not just silence important notions in biomedicine which are considered by members of this organisation to be unhelpful, but actively constructs an alternative way of seeing based on notions which are considered a more appropriate basis for working with the terminally ill.

18 According to Finkler (1991:76), these skills (which are based on a diagnostic process which identifies disease entities using universal nosological classifications), and treatments, are arguable the hallmark of biomedical activity (1991:76).

19 MacCormack notes that (1994:viii) 'medical students are still overwhelmingly rewarded for their ability to perform technical procedures, make diagnoses and prescribe curative therapies. The ability to just be present with another person is not overtly valued in the training process.' In relation to the use of technology, such training reinforces the physician's needs to get as much information as possible rather than a concern for the experience of being tested for the patient. Preston (1981:121) refers to this kind of behaviour as 'The doctor is treating himself (sic).'

20 Hart describes Biomedicine as driven by a technological determinism which is oriented towards the manipulation of organic symptoms with the intention of effecting their disappearance (if at all possible), and hence is primarily concerned with 'cure' rather than 'care'. Similarly, Hewa and Hetherington (1990:183) point to the devaluation of non-technologically oriented patient care work as characteristic of the scientific biomedical model that dominates medicine today.

21 This emphasis on technology is seen by Relman (1980:969) to lead to excessive fragmentation of care, overspecialism and overemphasis on expensive technology.

9 Coming into existence: the threats

> Not every group that attempted to create a hospice program succeeded. Hospice supporters claimed that hospice programs were a desired change; in actuality, there was a great deal of resistance to them. This resistance, however, never coalesced into formal attempts to stop the hospice movement (Siebold, 1992:105).

So far in this discussion, KHS has been shown to be a service with a difference: a difference based on notions of spirituality, holism, and choice. Such an alternative organisation, with its different 'way' of working with the dying would, according to the hospice literature, generally be seen as unlikely to succeed in establishing itself. The following discussion looks at what the data from this research had to say about this process of coming into existence.

Existence was far from assured

A foundational assumption for the following analysis is the understanding that, although KHS did manage to negotiate its existence, this was not inevitable. Local experience (Private Palliative Care Association) and the hospice literature (DuBois, 1980:131; Wilson, 1983:243) give ample evidence of attempts at hospice formations that were not successful. Such attempts were seen to fail because of factors they share in common with KHS's history, such as personality factors (Siebold, 1992:104-5), funding and professional support issues (DuBois, 1980:131), concerns about reliance on grant money, and hindrance because of the medical profession's inability to cope with issues of death and dying (Wilson, 1983:243).

To 'set the stage' for a full exploration of how KHS managed to negotiate its existence, it is important to look first, at what the participants had to say about factors (specific to KHS's development) which could have blocked its existence. The focus will then turn (in the following chapter) to an examination of how the embryonic organisation of KHS came to negotiate its existence in spite of such threats.

Siebold's 'impediments' to hospice growth

As outlined in the introductory quote of this discussion, Seibold acknowledges the actuality of substantial, though not formal, obstacles which characteristically offers a challenge to hospice development. These 'impediments' to hospice growth, as translated from Siebold's work (1992:124), can be summarised into three categories embracing funding, professional disapproval and concerns about the hospice discourse on dying. Such a classification resonates with the present findings and so will be used to organise the material for this discussion.

The problem of funding

Funding talk is central to understanding both the genesis and possible obliteration of the KHS project. As will be explored later, the nature of KHS's funding is seen as a Janus-headed influence, which takes whilst giving, imposes whilst empowering, and restricts whilst freeing. As a factor in determining the fate of KHS's bid for existence funding cannot be overstated. The seriousness of concerns about funding can be seen by one participant's comment as follows,

> We were within an inch of having to close our doors at one stage. If the department hadn't of come, we had to borrow about fifty or sixty thousand dollars to continue and that money ran out, and it is only government funding which has allowed us to grow and develop (EQ).
>
> ...unless you have a huge cash flow and we didn't have, as you probably know. If an accountant had looked at what we were starting with they would have just laughed and thrown it in the bin..I mean it was a fool's paradise (EQ).
>
> The main problem at the time was lack of money (EQ).

An inability or failure to arrange financial resources is recorded as the chief threat to hospice program implementation (Clark, 1993:176; Breindel and Boyle, 1979:43). Because the need for funding is so powerful, and the access to such finances so limited for most hospice projects, the search for this resource is seen to have a powerful impact on hospice independence (Siebold, 1992:107). According to Abel (1986:78), the direction KHS took to obtain funds, that is obtaining government support, was characteristic of hospice administrations. Indeed, such government support is now cited as evidence of hospice success and legitimation within the health care system (Greer et al., 1986:9). The rationale given by other hospices for seeking government monies, similar to KHS, is that other forms of fund raising are so time consuming, and thus divert too much time from other important tasks of the service.

Financial need translates into dependence on a more dominant discourse, especially if the funding body is a government agency who dictates the conditions under which monies are provided. Adaptation to such demands is seen to be characteristic of hospice formation: the very funding that is necessary for negotiating and sustaining existence brings with it conditions and demands that can also undermine the original ideals of the receiving service (ibid). Because funding is such a powerful issue and, in the case of this hospice, is linked into the hegemonic discourse of mainstream health, such a threat has a significant influence on organisational discourse. These ideas will be explored further later.

Professional disapproval

Siebold's second point concerning resistance to hospice formation was that of professional disapproval by physicians who saw hospice staff as 'morbid do-gooders' primarily preoccupied with notions of dying (1992:125).

Such professional disapproval was also indicated by participants, who mentioned nursing as well as physician criticisms of KHS's practices with the dying. Mention was also made of the risk health professionals took with their own reputation by becoming involved in KHS. The difficulty centred around KHS's early reputation as 'Just that bunch of Buddhists'.

As with funding, the threat of professional disapproval was a very powerful notion. Dependent on other professionals for referrals, support, and liaison KHS needed to resist being marginalised by mainstream health professionals. The extent to which this posed early problems is illustrated by the following comment from a participant,

> Because I think in the early days for a lot of those players, they actually had a bit at risk in being identified with Karuna. In fact, I can think of someone who was an early knocker of Karuna, this person now lives interstate..'Oh well, of course you know, I have my reputation and I would have to be very careful not to be identified with Karuna (EQ).

As will be discussed in the next chapter, resistance to such threats was built through the incorporation of high prestige/high profile professionals who secured a respectable standing for KHS. At the same time, members of the KHS team worked long hours and with great perfectionism to secure a name of high repute.

Such threats to professional standing did not just come from the gaze from without, but were also seen to be a function of problems associated with the early public discursive practices of KHS.

Seen to be 'flowering up palliative care', 'making palliative care more than it is', and 'promising the world and not delivering', such discursive practices alienated important individuals both outside and within KHS. According to Kane (1986:3) such a discourse of hyperbole is often associated with the introduction of new movements. The mentioned flowery speech about death can be interpreted as 'the need to sell innovative concepts by promising dramatic effects'.

The appropriate referrals from other health professionals working in the field is an essential element, not only in KHS's establishment but also in their ongoing existence. The threats to such a referral process were seen to be attitudinal, organisational, philosophical and political.

Some of the reasons forwarded by participants which interfered with appropriate referrals to KHS included hospitals lacking palliative care teams; inadequate patient discharge services; specialist territoriality; attitudinal problems at the interface of curative and palliative medicine; lack of knowledge of choice; the belief that patients cannot be managed at home; and personality problems. Such notions resonate throughout the hospice literature (Hyman and Bulkin, 1990; Gochman and Bonham, 1988; Munley, 1983:19; Cochrane et al., 1990). There are innumerable reasons provided by hospice research which reinforce this notion of professional resistance and they include such issues as scepticism from the medical community (Abel, 1986:76), the newness of the hospice concept, the negative images of death, the generalised avoidance of the dying and those who work with the dying (Levy, 1982:297), the denying and disguising of death throughout society (Farrell, 1982:120), the above average fear of death by physicians and their 'never say die' attitude which delays the transition palliative mode (Crowther, 1980:27), and the emphasis in medical training on cure (Corr and Corr, 1983: Siebold, 1992:152).

Understandably, 'death prior to admission', caused by delay of referral, has been recorded as the most important single reason for non-admission to hospice services (Creek, 1982:53; MacDonald, 1989:40). In terms of such research, KHS's experience of such resistance has been similar to most.

Concerns about the hospice discourse on dying

Siebold's third category of resistance from mainstream organisation to hospice development, which refers to hospice attitudes to death, focused on the issue of euthanasia. Interestingly, the topic of euthanasia was not raised, indeed, the word was never mentioned. However, there was an important attitudinal area of KHS's early work with the dying which was privileged as an important factor in creating resistance from both those inside and outside this organisation. This area of concern focuses on how the members of KHS's embryonic organisation refer to their experiences with the dying.

The resistance centred on the notion of unrealistic hyperbole about the experience of working with the dying, and concern about workers inappropriately 'getting off on death', rather than respecting the intensely personal nature of the experience. The workers who operated in this way were referred to as 'death and dying junkies'.

The literature on hospice care suggests a number of factors which can begin to build an understanding of such a phenomenon. A start would be with the very generalised notion of a 'good death' or 'death with dignity'. The KHS discourse is situated within the international hospice discourse of 'death with dignity'. Unfortunately, according to Martocchio (1982:15), there is no exact definition of this concept and so such a phrase can be interpreted to have many meanings. Such a notion of 'death with dignity' can be seen to incorporate a number of bipolar opposites ranging from for example, person/nonperson; self control/other control; or acceptance-peace/protest-rage. The point is, that interpretation of the concept is, particularly in the early stage of the hospice movement, very open to rhetoric and individual interpretation.

The literature also indicates that early enthusiasts in hospice care tended to have high aspirations based on a romantic view of human nature, and so consequently used superlatives in their descriptions of goals and experiences. In the words of Abel, such workers,

> Like many reformers they had a romantic view of human potential. They described death as a 'growth-filled event' and as being 'beautiful though sorrowful'. By providing 'an enabling and loving climate', some hoped to foster a new intimacy among family members. Others had even more grandiose expectations: they envisaged changing the directions of modern society, deflecting it from its obsessions with technological solution (1986:74).

Descriptives such as 'wonderful', 'beautiful' and 'glorious', which members of the embryonic KHS used to inscribe the dying experience, fit well into this discourse of the early hospice reformers.

However, the language texts suggest that more than just a descriptive process was at work in creating such criticism and resistance from others. There appeared to be psychological mechanisms at work, as inscribed by the idea of 'getting hooked on that experience'. For this reason, Pattison's work on professional distortions of denial of death (1977:15) will be used to provide further assistance in understanding this phenomenon. According to Pattison, the denial of death in health professionals can take contradictory forms of both detachment and exaggerated compassion. It is the second form which appears to have some relevance to this discussion. The psychological mechanism here is described as fusion with the patient's experience: the individual experiences an inability to differentiate self from others. The worker thus experiences afresh with each terminal patient, a dying and consequent rebirth. Described as a vicarious identification, the worker is seen to use the experience to undo past guilts, relieve past shame, restore personal self-esteem, or rework their own prior death experiences and anticipate their own death anxieties. An inbuilt psychological reward is the way in which the worker, unlike the patient, survives to rebirth and experiences a momentary victory over death. Such a process translates into professional over-involvement with patients. Psychologically and ethically, the worker's commitment has more to do with their own needs than that of their patients. This was hinted at in the language/texts by the following comments,

> I guess it is private and has to do with the person and it is not to do with you...you're there to support, you are not there to get off on it (EQ).

> Well, when someone continually talks about how wonderful the death was and what beautiful death someone had, and how glorious it was,... and continually it was like a high and that is what I am saying...it was like the person was being disregarded (EQ).

Such practices, understandably, were viewed as ethically unacceptable, and placed KHS open to the criticism and condemnation of the health professional community. These practices can be contrasted with the clear notion of the role of the health professional in a situation which privileges death with dignity, as described by Martocchio,

> To die a 'good death' or a 'death with dignity' involves dying with as much self control, privacy, comfort, attention, and support as dying persons desire and can achieve. It entails the dying persons' participating in decisions affecting them. It entails assistance and support. Hence, it is not a death dominated by others (1986:15).

This definition, interprets dignity as respect for individuals by support for their autonomous choice. Such an approach would not offer unrealistic notions which are impossible to realise, nor suppress the many difficult emotions surrounding dying that are important, but perhaps a little less acceptable. As Pattison suggests (1977:15), to acknowledge the universal ambivalence to dying, with all the emotions of anger, despair, frustration, disappointment and even hatred, is as important as any discourse which focuses on the feelings of tender, loving compassion.

There were ingredients, it is argued, in KHS's early discourse on working with the dying that were a threat to their credibility and thus existence.

Ego needs and the conflict of personalities

One threat to existence, which is not strongly privileged in the hospice literature, but which was considered to be of considerable importance to the participants, is that of the conflict of personalities.

Although often dealt with in the literature on stress and burnout, the notion of personality conflict was only referred to tangentially in the research on hospice formation. Hospice leaders may make passing remarks on the organisational tension generated by individual differences, such as 'If you don't have problems you don't have hospice' (Lamers, 1988:9), or 'If they don't have scars they haven't worked as a team' (Paradis, 1987), but this is usually in reference to team building, not threats to hospice existence. Perhaps one of the reasons for the silencing of such a notion could be the privileging of the positive, the harmonious, the compassionate 'we spirited' orientation to human relationships in hospice discourse (Munley, 1983:58). At the centre of the hospice discourse is an implied assumption that workers should be above such 'petty issues' and simply work for the 'good of the patient' (Paradis, 1987:151). Indeed, research indicates that a commitment to the 'good death' philosophy can cause stress and burnout because of unrealistic expectations such an ideal represents to workers. For such workers, the emphasis on high motivations and ideals is not balanced by a realistic appreciation of the human pressure of such a task (Jeffrey, 1993:32). Hospice workers can find themselves torn between a demanding ideology and demanding patients (Munley, 1983:206).

The readiness of the participants to privilege personality issues is thus not only considered a difference to what would be expected if reading the research material on hospice, but will also be sanctioned in this interpretation as a real strength of KHS's discourse. Whilst endorsing a 'gentle spirituality', this organisation also demonstrated, through the language/texts, a real ability to acknowledge issues of personality difference and tension.

Fairclough (1989:41; 1992:12) writes about the opacity of discourse (and practice in general), where particular power relations within organisations can be legitimated without members being consciously aware of the nature of such power or the individual 'will to power' behind such discursive practices. Members can use inspiring and emotive talk about the goals and activities of their organisation to disguise their own needs and ends. An important ethical aspect of studying discourse for Fairclough becomes that of raising people's consciousness so that individuals become aware of such power relations. With regards to KHS, however, the research data suggested that members were well aware of, and able to speak about, how their personal (ego) needs were being met (and perhaps disguised by) the inspirational mission of their organisation.

The language/texts are full of examples of discourse awareness and self-reflexivity [1] of the participants. There surfaced an awareness, not only of the differing ideological positions separate individual could take, but also of the nexus between an inspirational ideology and personality needs. The research participants inscribed, on many occasions throughout the interviews, an inner searching and a personal awareness of the relationship between their altruistic ideological beliefs about serving humanity and the individual satisfaction they were receiving from the experience. In short, participants demonstrated self-reflexivity and a high level of conscious awareness of the implications, both organisationally and psychologically, of their discursive practices. Some examples of this can be seen as follows,

> I like to think that I was coming from some greater force of wanting to benefit dying people, but at the end of the day it was about what I needed and I think that those who went there in the early days, it was about what they needed (EQ).

> The first ones (training courses) were very much ego driven like it was exciting, it was like we were really (pioneering, breaking new territory). Yes, so there was a lot of ego in it and I think for me there was a lot of excitement and a great sense of oh, this is something I really want to do, and the concept was unique. And there was also a sense of where was it going to go was it going to work or was it not going to work (EQ).

I think the ego has an attraction to saying I am doing something different..you don't even know you are doing it until you are actually there I was always attracted to the things that were different (EQ).

The very fact that such information surfaced and was offered freely is taken to be a sign of the high level of self-reflexivity KHS members bring to their understanding of organisational issues. Such discourse strengths can be seen as playing an important role in both negotiating with other organisations and in resolving conflict within the service. The privileging of notions of ego needs and conflict of personalities does not indicate that KHS had any more conflict than other organisations, or that such conflict was of a more severe threat to existence, but rather that the discursive practices of KHS were strong enough to accommodate such a fullness of discussion.

Such reflexivity is in character with the Buddhist ideological base which reinforces the importance of the individual's personal journey, and of the need for the individual to be aware of their own desires and intentions.

Conclusion

This discussion has outlined the notions which were recorded in the language texts, as to the perceived 'threats' KHS faced when coming into existence. Such factors were detailed using Siebold's analysis of 'impediments' to hospice growth (1992:124).

In the next chapter, the focus will turn to the many sociological and organisational factors which facilitated KHS's existence, in spite of such threats. The discussion will be concerned with privileging the positive influences which fostered success. Such a generic discussion will be concerned with macro-issues of genesis, and will be set within the literature on charismatic movements (James and Field, 1986), counter-institutions (Abel, 1986), and the hospice reform movement (Siebold, 1992).

Note

1 In this context self-reflexivity is a notion used in the literature on discourse which is similar (in some ways) to the idea of self-consciousness. To understand this notion it is important to first consider Davies (1994:19) insights into discourse when he states that 'the constitutive power of ways of talking and writing are not usually made visible. Rather, they are usually regarded as the transparent medium through which real worlds are described and analysed, real worlds which have their existence independent of the words spoken about them'. Self-reflexivity is then understood as the ways individuals within a discourse do make other realities visible. The example given in this text being that the members of KHS have the ability to break through the 'real world' of their spiritual discourse to acknowledge another world: that of the satisfaction of their own ego needs. In so doing they are displaying a degree of self-reflexivity.

10 Coming into existence: success

This chapter centres on exploring the process by which KHS successfully responded to and overcame the obstacles to establishing a service with a difference. The intent is to make a contribution to the international body of literature on hospice development through the local, ad hoc insights on KHS's formation.

As funding and legitimation had to come from the hegemonic discourse of biomedicine, the focus will remain at the interface between KHS and biomedicine. The discussion so far has highlighted the difference between these discourses. Indeed, part of the stated vision and value base of those initiating KHS was to develop this very difference. As will be seen through the following discussion, hospice projects that had the financial backing and professional support of the medical profession were seen to be most likely to succeed. The more alternative the option from conventional medicine, the less likely the project's survival. Indeed, Siebold records, community-oriented programs, such as KHS, with small, primarily volunteer staff had great difficulty surviving. They were without a strong political base, and so were not seen as an important part of the hospice movement (Siebold, 1992:138). The present discussion will explore the *contradiction* of an alternative discourse (KHS) which sets out to be *different* from mainstream health, but which, in doing so, establishes itself by building on its *similarities* to such a hegemonic discourse. KHS's alternative discourse will be exposed to reveal a conservative centre. By using Starr's notion (1979) of an 'exemplary counterinstitution', the silenced conservative notion in KHS's discourse will be uncovered. The reading (or interpretation of) this organisation's success then becomes predicated on this richer understanding of the contradiction or paradox of conservatism informing alternative resistance to hegemonic power.

Whilst engaging in this exploration of the genesis of KHS, the discussion will also begin to introduce and explore the other side of the contradiction of 'conservatism in difference' by looking at the 'difference in such sameness'. It will be argued that, although there are strong, conservative, conforming notions at the ideology-language interface of this organisation, this does not negate the possibility of a second level agenda of resisting whilst conforming. In the case of KHS, such resistance is attributed to the spiritual discourse; the very discourse responsible for energising and guiding the establishment of this service. The spiritual discourse, consequently, will be presented as a paradox: a discourse underpinned by conservative notions which actively facilitate its links with the hegemonic power of mainstream medicine, whilst at the same time providing the discursive space to assert a difference to the very discourse (biomedicine) which sustains it.

The beginning to this story is a group of visionaries in the community who voluntarily give of their time and effort for a dream about an alternative way of working with the dying. This initiative is neither physican-led, nor the outgrowth of hospital (tertiary care) planning. In short, the story begins well outside of the biomedical system. In the face of such odds, and in consideration of the already outlined threats to its existence, how then can KHS's survival be interpreted?

Overview

> Hospice growth and survival depends on its members' success in convincing other individuals and institutions to provide such resources as money, legal entitlements, and public support for its activities (Levy, 1982:294).

The story of KHS which unfolds in the statements of the participants is one of a strong charismatic leader, who is energised by a vision imparted by his Buddhist teacher and who brings together a network of dedicated and highly respected professionals and hard working volunteers. Through 'sheer blood sweat and tears' this group of volunteers eventually managed to negotiate KHS's existence by the establishment of an excellent reputation and public funding. As will be seen in the following discussion, such a story resonates with the hospice literature. The key ingredients which contributed to the successful outcome were seen to be: the charismatic leadership; the energy and dedication of its members; the shared vision and values; the links with mainstream health professionals and individuals in powerful positions; and the consequent successful attainment of legitimacy and hence funding. In short, KHS, like other successful hospice projects, managed to convince other individuals and institutions to provide the resources necessary for its existence, such as money, legal entitlements and public support.

An 'exemplary' counter-institution

> We wanted to start something that did have more of a people, community people, rather than institutional kind of base to it, and something that

would try and provide what people really needed themselves in order to care for someone (EQ).

Unlike other hospice experiments that start within the financial and professional power base of established medicine, KHS's attempt began in the community with a core of dedicated 'visionaries'. The individuals involved were described as 'a little non-mainstream', spiritually based people with an 'alternative' value system: 'people interested in Buddhism, other alternative ways, types of thought, people who took up meditation, yoga, all sorts of backgrounds' (EQ).

Their vision for starting 'Karuna' was described as the development of a community based, caring service for the dying which was based on a person-centred, compassionate approach: 'A shared dream, that we wanted to create something different...really wanted it to be whole' (EQ).

This resonates with Abel's description (1986:71) of the early leaders of the hospice movement, who shared a number of attitudes with the founders of the alternative institutions of the 1960s and early 1970s. These values included nostalgia for the simple ways of yesteryears, dissatisfaction with bureaucratic and authoritarian institutions, faith in the power of nature, a resistance to expert control, and a commitment to enhance the quality of personal relationships.

As outlined in the discussion on the description of KHS's difference, many of the spiritual and attitudinal values held both by the original and present members of KHS hinge on these concerns about simplicity, egalitarianism, holism, interdisciplinarity and the nurturing of relationships. 'A less institutional way of caring for people and a more person centred, caring compassionate, rather than a more institutional model'(EQ).

Consequently, the original visionaries of KHS will be seen to be holding the notions described by Starr (1979:245) as the 'romantic' ideal of the counterinstitution. Indeed, one participant made an explicit connection by pointing out that most of the individuals who have been involved in KHS would, because of the similarity of their present ages, have had their formative philosophical development during the what has now been colloquially described as 'the 60s'.

According to Starr (1979:246), there are two types of counterinstitutions: exemplary and adversary. The embryonic KHS, had many of the characteristics of the exemplary institution, described as,

> a utopian community .. (which) seeks, as the term suggests, to exemplify in its own structure and conduct an alternative set of ideals -the ideals, its organisers may hope, of a new society. Compared with established institutions, it may attempt to be more democratic in its decision-making, or less rigid and specialised in its division of labor.. its aim is the direct and independent realisation of its ultimate values, within the circumference of its own activities (1979:246-7).

The statements of members of KHS, whether they were articulating the original goals or presenting recent organisational ideals, were characterised by such idealistic, democratic notions: '(What they) didn't want was a whole lot of layers of people and kind of orders and differentiation' (EQ). The concern from the very start was to 'create an organisation that was different and not like hospitals' (EQ).

Such an 'exemplary' agenda differs markedly from that of the 'adversary' counterinstitution, which Starr describes as 'concerned with altering the prevailing social order' (1979:247). Many of the significant early leaders in hospice establishment, such as Dame Cecily Saunders, although acknowledging a sub-agenda of education through demonstration, explicitly stated their position as 'adversary': the central goal was to instigate mainstream reform (Fulton and Owen, 1981:173). Indeed, many authors, when referring to the sociology of hospice development, talk of the 'hospice movement', with its orientation to health care reform (Abel, 1986:81; Klagsbrun, 1981:18; MacDonald, 1990:40; Wald etal., 1980:173). In the words of James and Field, 'the hospice movement is unashamedly reformist' (1992:1363).

According to Abel (1986:81), the hospice movement grew out of a larger movement to humanise care for the dying, fostered by such pioneering leaders as Elizabeth Kubler-Ross. Early hospice leaders were seen to be incorporating ideas from diverse reform movements, such as holistic care, women's health, the home birth movement, and self-care, which challenged notions of medicalization, medicocentricism and the benefits of technology. Central issues for such reform movements were the demystification of medical knowledge, and the promotion of more equitable relationships between patients and physicians (ibid).

Dame Cecily Saunders, the acknowledged leader of the hospice reform movement, argued for the universal benefit for all patients of such compassionate care, whether or not in terminal stages of their disease. Her revolutionary vision of hospice development was that with the appropriate integration of palliative ideas within mainstream medicine, hospices could 'self-destruct' through obsolescence (Fulton and Owen, 1981:17). Such reform was seen to be revolutionising the health care system 'from the inside out' (Saunders, Summers and Teller, 1981:17).

How do the original and present goals and aspirations of KHS relate to such reformist notions? Could KHS be seen as a predominantly 'adversary' rather than an 'exemplary' institution?

One of the original, implicit assumptions that informed the development of this research was the belief that KHS's 'mission' was of a very alternative and challenging nature: perhaps similar to Starr's notion (1979:247) of an 'adversary' counterinstitution. Resistance was considered an important research topic because, by a process of linear reasoning, for an organisation to be alternative meant, *ipso facto,* for it to be a threat/challenge to mainstream. The radical character of the KHS agenda, by such reasoning, carried with it an implied notion that it would be a reforming organisation. Indeed, the whole notion of resistance was chosen for a research focus because this assumption engendered a curiosity about how such a powerless group of people could manage to challenge such a hegemonic discourse (biomedicine) and succeed in establishing itself.

By looking not only at what is being stated explicitly in this discourse (that is the alternative mission of establishing a very different approach to working with the dying) but also at what is being silenced (the similarity to many mainstream ideas), the data collected can be read to suggest that the 'alternative' discourse of KHS contains disguised conservative ingredients. On the exemplary/reform or radical/conservative continuum, KHS's agenda has many essential elements which fit comfortably with, and are an extension of, the professional mainstream health discourse. The discursive articulations of both the 'dream Karuna' and the spiritual orientation of many of its early and present members, although ostensibly widely different from mainstream health practices, are still, it is argued, conceptually conservative. Such conservatism is inherent in the desire expressed as a 'will to serve' as opposed to what would be a more radical desire of the 'will to destroy and recreate'.

KHS's 'difference', thus, may not be as radical as first appears, if the pragmatic goal of starting KHS are examined closely. 'And that common goal is to help people, with however you define helping' (EQ). Descriptions of such a goal were couched in words such as to 'serve', 'help', or to 'care', with the intent of bringing a '...spiritual interest into helping others in a very practical way' (EQ). In the words of one participant,

> Each one had a selfless motivation...and willing to serve others, and a willingness to make great sacrifices, personal sacrifices to serve others and I think historically that has always been a great ingredient for success (EQ).

Certainly, the agenda and rhetoric of many mainstream health care professionals and organisations is also to serve, help and care. As explained by Abel (1986:81), although hospice development has its roots in progressive reform movements, there are also many conservative elements. Indeed, the leader of this organisation clearly stated a wish to affirm the link, and therefore the similarity, with similarly minded carers, be they professional or voluntary, within the bio-medical system, when he stated,' I just see it as being a group of ordinary committed people who are trying to offer a compassionate service and compassion is something universal and it is practised all over the world' (EQ).

Thus, by analysing the KHS discourse it is apparent that there are many conservative elements which share a commonality with the ways of speaking in mainstream health care institutions. The KHS discourse may be a discourse of resistance, it may be a well articulated alternative to mainstream health care with the dying, it may be a compassionate and caring response to the problems people face with terminal illness, but that does not necessarily mean that it incorporates a challenging reform agenda. Abel (1986:81) attributes much of the reason for the increased popularity of the hospice movement to simultaneous appeal to both progressives and conservatives. KHS, it has been argued, is seen to contain such a dual appeal.

While some may question that there is a radical reform agenda based upon particular interpretations of the discourse used, this is not to argue, by polar opposites, that KHS was *no* threat to established institutions. There were, indeed, factors attributed specifically to KHS's difference (such as its Buddhist underpinnings and its initial inexperience in the hospice area of work) which created resistence. As well as this, as Wald and associates argue (1980:175), there are notions inherent in hospice philosophy that are a 'challenge to the status quo'. A focus on palliative treatment for control of symptoms challenges the curative orientation to do battle at all costs. Compassionate, intensive personal care for the patient and family may not be compatible with intensive technology. Family participation is a challenge to institutional routines. Interdisciplinary teams, with strong nurse management, are a challenge to medical specialisation. Continuity of care challenges the territoriality of multiple health agencies operating separately.

Whilst the early members of KHS, in order to establish their service, needed to negotiate with the hegemonic power of the biomedical system,[1] conservative notions inherent in their ideology facilitated such resistance. If viewed as an 'exemplary counter-institution', non-reformist, conservative ingredients in their ideology provided a protective, adaptive element to their discursive practices which deflected, to some extent, the full power of the system. The task of the founding members was to initiate a service, to gain legitimacy, to establish funding, and to develop working relationships with other health professionals in the area. Their goals were service oriented, and local. Whilst other early hospice leaders wanted no less than to revolutionise the health care system (Saunders, Summers and Teller, 1981:17), or to change the direction of modern society away from its obsession with technological solutions (Abel, 1986:74), the founding members of KHS were 'visionaries' with a 'will to service' and a more modest agenda of service provision. The words used to express their vision were those of creating, of compassion, of caring, of helping. Notions of challenging, destroying, or reforming, were not privileged.

As will be later explored, KHS followed the predicted trajectory of exemplary institutions. Once it managed to survive more than a few years, and secured the necessary resources from the established order, then, with respectability gained, it began to risk becoming more like the biomedical institutions it originally sought to differ from (Abel, 1986:83). Most medically-funded hospices come to be indistinguishable from mainstream organisations: a point of ongoing concern for the present members of Karuna.

So far, it has been argued, that KHS began with a discourse of co-optation, not confrontation, and this has direct relevance in understanding notions of establishment /resistance.

Creating the links

> Hospices and earlier counter-institutions also faced similar problems. Although they originally sought to provide alternatives to the established order, they were forced to rely on mainstream institutions for resources, political acceptance, and personnel. Integration, in turn, compelled them to modify their practices and goals (Abel, 1986).

Links with mainstream funding, political power, and professionals had to be created and fostered.[2] To come into existence, early members of KHS needed to establish funding, arrange for patient referrals, build relationships with other health professionals, and gain the confidence and respect of public and health professionals working in the area.

Although not out to reform or attack mainstream practices with terminal patients, the Buddhist based, spiritual agenda of this group of 'visionaries' was seen as sufficiently 'different', to create resistance. Consequently, the embryonic organisation was marginalised as 'Just that bunch of Buddhists': a term perceived as a derogatory attack on their professional credibility and the legitimacy of their work in the area of palliative care. Coming into existence, and maintaining resistance has, for this organisation, necessitated both developing the essential resources needed to run the service, as well as establishing a respectable reputation as a credible alternative in the area of hospice/palliative care.

Throughout the following detailed examination of this process, three key factors will be highlighted as operating in KHS's discursive practices at its genesis. The first is the significant role of the charismatic leadership as an ingredient to the success of this organisation. The second, is the leader's consciously conceived and active process of incorporating or co-opting, from the very beginning, high profile professionals who bring dedication and skills. The third is a process, expressed in lay terms as 'preaching to the converted', in which the discursive practices of this organisation attract others with similar patterns of talk, or ways of being. In such a 'pioneering' organisational project, the discursive power to attract 'like-minded' individuals is as important in resistance as is any proselytising notion of domination.

An examination of the above issues will begin by focusing on the notion of charismatic leadership.

Charismatic leadership

> But I have a great deal of respect for him...he is a very charismatic person and he can get people very motivated and very involved...what he is good at doing is...dreaming and he is good at putting those sort of things into place (EQ).

> He has been the linchpin right through and I have heard a lot of people say that if (he) leaves Karuna, Karuna won't be the same (EQ).

The participants clearly saw the original director to be a charismatic leader, the moving force behind the establishment of the KHS. It was this charismatic leader's dream, his ability to motivate and include others, his integrity and his energy which are seen as central factors in the successful process by which KHS was brought into existence. As one participant summed up the situation, 'Karuna could not have happened without him...I am sure...with his ability to attract people with expertise and people with drive...I mean he was very much a driving force' (EQ).

This notion of a charismatic leader as the instigator and moving force behind hospice creation resonates with the hospice literature. According to Levy (1982:300), hospice formation typically begins from the idea of a single, interested individual. From there, the idea spreads according to the individual's ability to convert others to the vision. Historical accounts thus record the personal influence of a strong, charismatic leader as a usual or likely antecedent of hospice formation. KHS's hospice formation fits this pattern of development from the genesis of an idea to the gathering together of a following.

The participants referred to the time of the idea formation for the hospice as the period of 'dreaming'.[3] This is an interesting metaphysical idea, which is not acknowledged in the hospice literature. Such a notion will be mentioned in the final chapter on future research agendas, as it appears to be a rich and constructive idea which could further our understanding of the human process/potential to create. The dream for KHS, the kernel of the idea, was stated by many of the participants to have come from their charismatic leader, as evidenced by the following transcripts,

> So we got to know (leader) quite well and he started to share this instruction he had got from (his teacher) and his dream..so we got involved with (him) and his dream (EQ).

The dream and the vision was described as being formalised by the request of the leader's Buddhist teacher. Although it must be noted that there were other key players, a nurse in particular, who shared that dream from the beginning, it was this spiritual leader who was seen as the central charismatic figure. Whether or not the leader was the only one with the original idea, the language/texts indicate that he is seen as the most significant of the original 'dreamers'. His ability to implement that dream through a consciously conceived, single minded plan of actively enlisting the support, skills and energy of many resourceful individuals was legendary to those who were members of, or associated with, this service. The early and conscious awareness of such a process can be seen clearly from his own words,

> From my side there is always the understanding, the perception, in order to be accepted and be successful and get support that we have to be very professional, we have to associate ourselves with people in the community who were respected and professionals, so then, in the early stage from the start (EQ).

Not only were such professionals seen as bringing reputations of note but also the valuable contribution of skills and resources. This leader's 'concept has always been to bring more and more skilled people into Karuna: it is like the saying the whole is greater than the sum of the parts' (EQ).

This process was described as an active one of seeking out the assistance of professionals that the developing service needed. In the words of the leader this process involved 'a combination of attracting those people, and also going out and seeking those people, and part of that has been the recognition of say weakness or areas within our service that needed to be developed' (EQ).

Equally, this process was acknowledged and affirmed by the other participants, who indicated that, 'he cleverly seconded a lot of people from a lot of different avenues of life and with a lot of different skills and connections and contacts and pulled them altogether..he got really hooked into people's dreams' (EQ).

Thus, it is argued that KHS, along with other successful hospice projects around the world, was realised through the driving force of a charismatic leader, capable of energising significant others to participate in his dream. This story fits well within the descriptions of pioneering-missionary organisations of hospices, which are initiated by natural leaders with charismatic authority who manage to inspire a following of committed workers (James and Field, 1986:1366-7; Punch, 1974:318; Wald et al., 1980:173). The task of charismatic leadership in the early stages of hospice formation is, according to Munley (1983:296), to inspire hope and confidence and to forge a dream that would attract a committed following. The transcripts of this research certainly privileges such a notion. Research indicates that this early inspirational role of the leader is, once the hospice is established, typically challenged by the need for administrative, managerial and organisational skills (Munley, 1983:296). As will be outlined in a later discussion, KHS follows this pattern.

Early hospice leaders, the most notable of whom was Dame Cecily Saunders, were characterised by their 'spirituality', their singleness of vision, intensity of purpose and narrowness of focus (James and Field, 1986:1367). In the published accounts of leaders such as Saunders, Wilkes, Doyle and Cassidy, a strong 'spiritual' influence is recorded: their power to engender enthusiasm in followers and to stimulate change being linked to their single-minded spiritual devotion to what they were doing (James and Field, 1986:1366). Indeed, research indicates that many involved in hospice referred to their work as a calling, with religious beliefs, predominantly Christian, underlying their philosophy of care for the individual. Others, though not professing a religious orientation, are documented as bringing a 'spirituality' or articulated philosophy of practice which gave meaning to life, death and suffering (Vachon, 1986:77).

Similarly, the charismatic leader of KHS openly acknowledged his debt to spiritual guidance. Unlike many of the other hospice leaders who have a Christian background, this leader follows a Buddhist metaphysic. This leader, understandably contributes the success of KHS to such spiritual inspiration and guidance. The inspiration and spiritual guidance of Lama Zopa Ripoche and his holiness the Dalai Lama, the power of prayer, the blessings of highly realised beings, and the compassion of all the Buddhas and Buddha saints were factors seen by this leader to be key ingredients in KHS's success.

Charismatic leadership is seen to be inherently unstable, resting to a large degree on the ability of the leader to generate and sustain support, which depends on the follower's belief and interest in the leader and his/her mission (James and Field, 1986:1366). The transcripts of this research strongly privilege the notion of this charismatic leader's early and ongoing support from his followers, as seen by the following comments,

> His mere presence with this team, has a most Rogerian, sort of non-directive person, he is very strong, people look up to him (EQ).

> The spiritual overseer of it all, and I think we all realise that it was his dream...his direction (EQ).

> I have nothing but respect for him and I have seen him just about walk through water almost to do what he thinks needs to be done, and to care about the place...he is on to being the greatest benefit to human beings (EQ).

> The most spiritual person I have ever met (EQ).

It has been argued that the key ingredient in the KHS discourse of its genesis has been the contribution of charismatic leadership, situated within the motivating and supportive metaphysical discourse of Buddhism. This leadership, it has been shown, was not only the initial catalyst to action, but also succeeded in activating and sustaining the ongoing support and motivation of followers for the establishment of this project.

Authors such as James and Field (1986) situate the analysis of hospice development within Weber's view of history. Weber's analysis acknowledges the possibility (as one among many factors) of exceptional individuals or charismatic leaders to act as catalysts of change: the power of the personal response to dissatisfaction with human circumstances (Bendix, 1966). However, Weber argues, such individual action, once institutionalised, gives way to bureaucratisation and rational socialisation (Bendix, 1966:326). History, according to Weber, alternates between charisma and rountinization through bureaucracy.

This research does not seek to universalize Weber's grand theory of social change. However, when contextualised to the local, ad hoc analysis of KHS, such analysis does contribute, to some degree, to an understanding of the phenomenon of resistance and the coming into existence of this organisation. James and Field (1986), applying Weber's theory to hospice development, articulate four key elements of charisma relevant to the early development of the hospice movement.

> The role of Cecily Saunders as a highly visible leader; the spiritual 'calling' which inspired many to become involved with hospices; the hospice vision of terminal care with its narrowness of focus; and the oppositional stance of the movement to mainstream terminal care (1992:1365).

All but the last of these key elements have already been discussed under the rubric of charismatic leadership. Parallels between such theory and the experience of KHS have been drawn. The last category of an 'oppositional stance' has tangentially been dealt with under 'exemplary counterinstitutions'. Although the leader of this project is, to some degree, a high profile public figure in the area of hospice/palliative care, neither he nor his followers, had an agenda of 'disruption or implied criticism' (ibid). Whilst acknowledging that even to create by example is, to some degree, to challenge the legitimacy of mainstream practice, it is argued that to see the project of KHS as 'oppositional' and 'disruptive' is problematic, and thus not sanctioning, to a sufficient degree, the conservative elements evident in this discourse of change. In this particular case, to affirm Weber's view that charismatic leaders are 'creative and disruptive' would be believed to overstate the radical/reform agenda of the formative members of this organisation.

The findings of this research affirm the usefulness of Weber's[4] analysis of the contribution of charismatic leadership. A caveat to such acknowledgment is the variability to the generic process demonstrated by an understanding of the development of this local, ad hoc project.

The people factor

> While such individuals can sustain the internal structure of a movement through their personality and efforts, these elements are seldom sufficient to override external opposition. To successfully push for hospice implementation, individuals must also hold prestigious or powerful positions outside the movement to give force and legitimacy to their demands. As one hospice organiser explained: 'The ideal person is a physician, the second is a strong likeable nurse, after that a minister or chaplain. If you don't have someone respected by the system, no one is going to listen to you' (Levy, 1982:300).

As already outlined in the section on charismatic leadership, the founding members of this service were very conscious of the sort of ideas Levy stated as the *modus operandi* for obtaining legitimacy. Through the two way process of both attracting and seeking the skills of high profile professionals, this organisation was seen to 'buy its legitimacy' (EQ) with mainstream organisation. Such a social practice is further evidence of the conservative underpinning of this 'alternative' discourse, which incorporated, from an early stage, many mainstream professional notions, such as, the prestige gained from educational qualification; the links between high profile professional reputations and establishing important connections with the wider health community; a respect for expertise; and an appreciation of the importance of well developed skills in providing a quality service. As an 'exemplary', rather than 'adversary', counter-institution, with a discourse that embraced notions of service, dedication, commitment, love, compassion, and holism; for many of the health professionals who became involved, the embryonic KHS discourse would, in many ways, have seemed an idealised extension of some of the rhetoric of their own professional subculture. This would be especially so if such professionals were already interested in hospice/palliative care issues.

There was, to some degree, a commonality of discourse, a sharing of respect for privileging the same notions of the power of prestige and the need to incorporate care as a central ingredient in service provision. From an early stage there is evidence of this discursive co-adaptation with mainstream service providers.

This is not to argue that there were no areas of resistance, or to suggest a sense of an accommodating mainstream bio-medical discourse ready to welcome the advent of an innovative hospice project. Indeed, as the literature suggests, initial resistance was to be expected, particularly in the form of scepticism from the medical community wary of any hospice project (Abel, 1986:76). Participants have outlined several important areas where resistance was felt and counter action was needed to assert and maintain their position. The chief points of resistance were stated to centre on the Buddhist nature of the organisation, the need to become more professional in palliative care skills, the difficulties experienced negotiating with general practitioners, and problems of referrals from mainstream institutions. Long term members of KHS recorded the early sense of 'scepticism' and implied criticism from other professionals working in the area, and the resultant 'need to prove themselves'.

> I mean our label was 'Oh that bunch of Buddhists'. Who do they think they are, what do they know, and so very much we were trying to say, 'we may happen to be a bunch of Buddhists, but we also happen to have these other skills and this great wish to serve and this ability to do things well'. So we spent a lot of time living down 'that bunch of Buddhists tag' (EQ).

The response to such implied criticism was hard work and dedication to service, developing a reputation based on excellence and competence, including people of high level skills and standing, developing links with people in power, maintaining an open attitude to learning whilst going along, and retaining a willingness to ask for advice. The hospice literature suggests such tactics are standard practice in the successful development of hospice projects.

Cherry (1982:313) clearly states that the incorporation of very high calibre team members is probably the most important reason for the success of hospices in both Britain and the United States. Possessing sufficient expertise to be credible, and stacking advisory boards with well-known and highly respected members whose names and credentials lend credibility to the project, such tactics are recorded as common strategies to overcome resistance and gain legitimacy (Munley, 1983:294; Levy, 1982:301). Prestigious and powerful individuals who understand the working of mainstream power structures have been recorded as the key ingredients in the success of hospice projects (Wald et al., 1980:177). According to Seibold (1992:116), political opportunity led to hospice proliferation.

In many ways, it can be seen that overcoming resistance to KHS's difference was for the members of KHS to become more like mainstream professionals. Resistance was not to accentuate the difference, but rather to affirm the similarity. Here, as elsewhere, the emerging discourse of KHS's evolution was one of co-adaptation to the demands, or 'will to power', of mainstream biomedicine. The 'struggle' was to prove competence in the hegemonic discourse of professionalism and skill, and not to challenge the very notions supporting such ideas of professional dominance.

Personal qualities, often described in such terms as 'dedication, 'commitment', 'energy', 'enthusiasm', 'experience', 'respect', 'talented', 'intelligent', 'hard working', and 'articulate', were also seen as key ingredients to KHS's success. Such attributes were seen as personal qualities of the individual professional /worker /volunteer. Such qualities combined with hard work and dedication, the belief that KHS's success was possible, a willingness to ask for advice, perfectionism, the joy of the work, shared goals and values, and the stability and quality of the individuals on the board, were seen to generate a powerful human dynamic of energy and commitment that established KHS's credibility and reputation. Such factors, it must be noted, are equally affirmed and privileged as positive by mainstream professionals. Participants comments on the workaholic aspect of KHS could equally be read as referring to the experience of many professionals within mainstream health organisation.[5]

A discourse that attracts

> The data suggest that hospices do not attract patients and families who demand aggressive, curative treatment beyond a reasonable hope of recovery. It would appear instead that hospice appeals to a discrete subset of the terminally ill population: namely patients and families who desire low-tech, home based care, an active role in care planning, and spiritual/emotional support in dealing with impending death, and for whom pain and symptom control, rather than protracted, curative struggle, is the primary concern (MacDonald, 1989:40).

One reading of the discussion so far could suggest that there is a one-way dynamic by which members of KHS actively seek out and incorporate the contribution of like-minded individuals. The impression that this was a small group of alternative 'visionaries' isolated from, but engaging in, building links with mainstream organisations, could be gained. However, the language/texts suggest a far more complicated process.

KHS's 'talk' and ways of being, attracts members and clients who share a similar world view. Like a discursive magnet, the KHS discourse drew into its circle of influence, professionals, volunteers, workers, clients and mainstream administrators eager to share its work and happy to contribute long hours and important skills to help create its success. Described by one participant as 'preaching to the converted', many of the key ingredients which facilitated KHS's existence, such as human resources and funding, were offered to, rather than actively sought out by, this organisation. Participants suggested that something in the 'very existence' of KHS 'vibrates' and offers something that seems to 'hook certain people'. KHS was not seen as a proselytising organisation, out to convert others to their ways of thinking, but rather one which 'preaches to the converted' and has its 'own sort of energy' which attracts those already interested in their philosophical base. The spiritual dimension was seen to be an important factor in attracting people to the work of KHS.

The web of relationships through which KHS negotiated its existence can thus be seen as a cycle of both attraction and engagement. The discourse, which alienates important members of this organisation, equally attracts and energises key figures within the network of significant relationships. By not attempting to be all things to all people, by accepting their difference with comfort, the members of KHS built much of their resistance, not by challenging those who disagreed, but by affirming the links with those who were sympathetic.

Parallel to this process, the members of the emerging KHS invest considerable energy into developing constructive community links through education and public speaking. As will be seen by the following discussion, there already was, however, a growing awareness of, and readiness to accept, the emerging ideas of hospice within the broader community.

The broader social context

> Charismatic movements can only be 'successful' if they resonate with tensions and ambiguities in the broader social context within which they arise (James and Field, 1986:1363).

Participants expressed the belief that there were attitudinal factors operating within society at the time of the formation of this service, that were instrumental in facilitating its development, such as the prevailing attitude in society for people to die at home and the contribution of professional conferences.

Such a notion is backed up by the literature on hospice development, as demonstrated by the following observation by Greer,

> Hospice arrived at the right time. Kubler-Ross had brought death 'out of the closet' and had spread discontent with the formalised impersonal bureaucratic system which, she said, was created for 'processing' the masses without consideration of the needs of individual patients. The 'right to die' and to control the manner of one's death was widely proclaimed. Professionalism, authoritarianism and advanced technology were under attack. Disillusionment with 'big' government and 'big' medicine were widespread (1985:82-3).

The ground work for such attitudinal change was attributed to such authors as Fiefel, Kubler Ross, Saunders and Mount, who incorporated ideas with practical experience (Wald et al., 1980:174). Mor and associates (1988:247) add to this list of attitudinal changes or social forces that generated the hospice movement, notions of vigorous and public opposition to 'extraordinary' interventions for the prolongation of life, the growth of home and community-based care, including the massive deinstitutionalization programs in the mental-health field, concerns about the rising costs of health care, particularly hospital costs, and the growth in popularity of 'alternative' practitioners. Such notions are backed up by other hospice/palliative care researchers (Field and James, 1993:7; Munley, 1983:295).

According to Wald and associates (1980:173), the last two decades have seen an increasing public awareness of issues related to death and dying, with open public discussion of the universal nature of the dying experience, and the implications of treatments and care for both the family and the patient.

Some authors, such as Field and James, record that the opportunity to die at home, comfortably in one's own bed, in the familiar surroundings of home with family and friends in attendance, as being seen by many to be the preferable or ideal way to die (1993:15). Hospice leaders articulated and furthered this growing community awareness. Other authors, such as Siebold (1922), however challenge this notion in relation to ideas of home being the place to die. Siebold, argues that hospice leaders used this romantic notion that there was a groundswell support for dying at home as part of their rhetoric, when in fact 'the public did not clamour for hospice services; rather, a minority constituency perceived that such a service was desirable' (Siebold, 1992:81). Hospice leaders would consequently be seen very much in the role of proselytising, rather than just responding. Certainly, it has not been my experience, as a palliative care educator, that there is, either with health professionals or the lay public, any generalised acceptance of or interest in issues of death and dying.

As discussed previously in the section on 'exemplary counter institutions', such discursive ideas on dying married well with the notions central to the counter institutional ways of seeing of the 1960s/70s. Modern, technologised death, in such a discourse, was the result of the 'course of nature' being ignored or distorted through excessive interventions of heroic life-saving techniques (Abel, 1986:73).

The members of the embryonic KHS chose to incorporate this recent discourse on death and dying (death-with-dignity and the right to die at home) into their discourse of genesis. These new discourse practices, idealised notions at the interface of language and hospice ideology, may or may not have reflected popularist beliefs, but were, in any case, an essential ingredient in developing a discourse of resistance. Studies certainly indicated, however, that in twentieth century industrialised societies, the great majority of the population were dying in hospitals and nursing home institutions, which is argued, by writers in the field of death and dying, to be not conducive to a peaceful and personalised death (Fulton, 1972). As has already been indicated in previous chapters, Australia is not an exception to such a trend (Kellehear, 1990:12). Research by Towsend and associates (1990:415) indicated that, with limited increase in community care, about 50% more patients with cancer could be supported to die at home as they and their carers preferred.

One of the few large scale studies of hospice outcomes indicates that the social practice of such discourses is effective in achieving the desired results of decreased use of technology with the dying and the possibility of allowing an increasing number to die at home. The National Hospice Study, USA, reported that hospice patients were less likely to receive therapies such as chemotherapy, surgery, radiation therapy, transfusions and intravenous therapy, and home care hospice patients spent more time at home (Mor et al., 1988). There is evidence that hospice discourse translates into practical ends deemed desirable by the discourse on 'death with dignity'.

There thus appears to have been sufficient support from many different social movements which would favour the formation of hospices. According to Munley (1983:295), one response to the discontent expressed in these alternative discourses of dissatisfaction with the dehumanising, but dominant, models of terminal care was the perception that hospice could do something better. Certainly, during this time, world-wide, there was a rapid proliferation of hospices, in diverse forms (Abel, 1986:74).

Several participants not only acknowledged the influence of these social movements, but also actively integrated such ideas through attendance at conferences, or visits to other model institutions. According to Siebold (1992:108), this was part of a world-wide trend towards conference attendance and publication, where participants endeavoured to learn more about the concept of hospice care. It became the practice of local initiators of hospice projects to consult the already existing models of hospices (James and Field, 1986:1367). KHS's efforts to come into existence must be set within the context of this international awakening of the need for the articulation of a discourse on hospice/palliative care.

Identifying the gap

To summarise, it has been argued that the process of facilitating KHS's negotiation/resistance rests on a janus-headed orientation of responding to the demands and criteria of mainstream health, whilst simultaneously being energised and supported by a spiritual discourse which attracts 'like-minded', dedicated individuals, who are committed to the 'cause' of working compassionately with the dying. Such a process, however, would not have sufficed in itself, without one very important ingredient, and that was the community need for such a service. The genius of KHS's founding members, it will now be argued, was expressed not only through their successful process of discursive negotiation but, as importantly, in their ability to listen to the needs of others and translate cries for help into service provision. In short, they shared the gift of being able to identify and respond to a significant gap in community services for the dying. This 'gap', this need, the *sine qua non* of KHS's evolution, was a determining influence in this organisation's development, from the very beginning, as the following statement indicates,

> Karuna would never have happened if there hadn't been a need. There were like these two conditions, there was this group of people who wanted to do it, but there was also this gaping need. And one without the other it

would never have happened (EQ).

An appreciation of the depth of such need was gained through the professional networks of the early players, who engaged in innumerable conversations with patients in the service organisations they were working for at that time, in particular through nursing contacts and a physiotherapy clinic. The dynamic of active listening, and the logistics of the sheer numbers (described as 'hundreds and hundreds of people') involved in the process can be seen by the following language/text,

> I think really it was just a matter of people kept coming into our circles who kept saying look, we need such and such, why don't you exist..for instance... physiotherapy clinic people would come to things like relaxation classes at this multidisciplinary clinic and they would talk about their problems and others they have to do with 'I can't find this' or 'I can't get that', 'why isn't there someone I can talk to', 'why doesn't anyone want to talk about death and dying'..so it was this identified sort of need, that people kept saying that you have always been very interested in death and dying so why don't you put something up, because you know we need it out there (EQ).

Such a process resonates in the literature on hospice development. Dame Cecily Saunders, the acknowledged originator of the hospice concept, describes a similar process as informing the formation of St Christopher's Hospice in London. For Saunders, 'it was not so much the general social trends, as the impact of listening to individual patients' that was the impetus for her work. This is similar to other hospice pioneers (Saunders, personal communication, 1991, cited in James and Field, 1986:1363-4). As demonstrated throughout this discussion, KHS's story of genesis is very similar to other hospice pioneers described within the literature.

The central point of this discussion then, is that the process of becoming, for KHS, as with other hospices world wide, rests not only on the effective negotiation of dominant discourses, but also on the accurate identification of a community discourse on the need for such practices. A driving force behind KHS's genesis, it is argued, is not only a spiritual motivation, but a clear perception of an expressed community need. Consequently, the discursive practices of KHS rest on an element of community development ideology, as expressed by one participant,

> This is a true community development in the purest sense, it was and that is why I was saying to him, this isn't something we have just dreamed up, we wouldn't have any clients, we wouldn't be getting donations, we wouldn't be getting help from anybody if people really didn't believe in us (EQ).

Such words inscribe not only a perception of unmet need, but also an awareness of being 'believed in', of being capable of meeting such expressed needs. These words hint at the conservative values underpinning much of

KHS's discourse of genesis, and this is the drive for legitimacy: the desire to be seen as 'as good as' other health professionals working with the dying.

Ruminations on spirituality

So far in this discussion, in an attempt to describe the different variables in this organisation's formation, a simplistic, one-sided picture of the members of KHS has been drawn. The conservative notions in KHS's alternative, 'exemplary' ideology has been revealed, and the similarity drawn to the dedicated, hard working and compassionate health professional in mainstream medicine.[6] In short, the compatibility with the hegemonic discourse of mainstream health professionals has been inscribed. Spirituality has only been mentioned tangentially.

In this discussion, emphasis has been placed on the texts which privilege the role of the high profile, professional individual with respect and contacts, in KHS efforts of resistance. *Such a story is paradoxical if viewed in terms ofthe original dreaming of this organisation.* The embryonic KHS fitted into Abel's description of hospice founders (1986:76) by being determined to start afresh, unencumbered by the practices, traditions and regulations of the traditional health care system: The vision was that dying 'could be really personal and intimate and nice and out of the medical model so that death took on more a part of life' (EQ).

In view of the present discussion of this organisation's strategies for accommodation, such goals appear to be compromised at best, a contradiction at worst. This contradiction will be addressed in the following two chapters which will explore the notion that the spiritual discourse running through KHS provides a degree of resistance to the hegemonic domination of mainstream health: the ideological *paradox of difference within sameness.* It will be argued that, although there are strong conservative and conforming notions at the ideology-language interface of this organisation, this does not negate the possibility of a second-level agenda of *resisting, whilst conforming*, through the spiritual dimension.

It appears superficially as if KHS submitted totally to the control and surveillance of the 'experts' of the dominant discourse. Although this happened to a large degree, there are ingredients within the spiritual discourse of KHS which keep resistance alive and offer the service and individuals working within it, some space to oppose the dehumanising influence of 'the system'. The postmodern notion of resistance, it must be stressed, is seen to be an ongoing and pervasive phenomenon. According to Fox (1993:57), resistance is ubiquitous and unexceptional, primarily achieved through local, everyday narratives and discursive practices.

The very fact that KHS successfully negotiated its existence may provide the vehicle, the discursive space, the compassion and caring necessary for local, ad hoc pockets of resistance to dehumanising influences of 'the system'. Spirituality, viewed in terms of postmodern notions of resistance, may in fact be *the* ingredient of actual resistance. Such a notion was privileged by the participants, as will be outlined in a later chapter.

No notion of understanding KHS's success or existence can avoid an appreciation of the powerful contribution of their spiritual discourse. As will be discussed in a later chapter, KHS's discourse creates a subjectivity and develops a working ethos which supports a positive spiritual orientation both at the organisational level and in work with their clients. This spiritual dynamic is not only a motivating force which has contributed to KHS's success, but, more importantly in terms of the present discussion, is the point of difference which embraces the *paradox of achieving alternative ends through a conservative discourse*.

Legitimacy gained

> (We) get quite a few referrals from hospitals..now receive government funding and we have proved ourselves (EQ).

KHS, like similar 'exemplary counterinstitutions', eventually gained the respect and support of mainstream organisations. The funding and referrals obtained from such support further secured this organisation's existence.

According to Levy (1982:295), all hospices, regardless of their organisational form, must forge and maintain reciprocal relations with existing medical authorities if they are to obtain funding and realise their organisational goals. Gaining funding from the Regional Health Authority was seen as a most important moment in the history of KHS's establishment as a hospice service. Good health economics and KHS's reputation for quality care were seen as the variables which convinced the Health Department of the benefits of funding this service. As finances had nearly run out at the time of funding, the state approved monies were seen to be THE most important factor in ensuring KHS's existence. The only other source of income was from donations, but this was not sufficient to run the service.

Similar again to the hospice literature, there are stated to be only two predominant ways such projects are funded: through government funding and charitable donations (Clark, 1993:170). Public financing is given as an important factor in the rapid proliferation of hospice services (MacDonald, 1990:40). With the exception of Hospice, Inc., in America, there are very few examples of successful hospices that managed to maintain their existence without public funding (Siebold, 1992:97-100). Thus, the story of KHS is characteristic of hospices worldwide.

As will be examined in more detail later in this work, such public funding led to many organisational tensions, whilst the members of this service negotiated the control and surveillance which comes as the down side of state monies.

As with funding, the establishment of a flow of referrals from mainstream health organisation and from professionals is also seen by members of this organisation as a sign of legitimacy.

> The people who refer to us...are referred by people who are accepting of

us...you know they don't say go see Karuna if they don't really agree with what we are doing (EQ).

Building up a reputation for excellence in the hospice field, engaging in educational and public speaking activities, contacts through satisfied clients, and a sympathy to KHS's philosophy on the part of the referring physician were all seen as important factors in gaining referrals from mainstream health professionals.

As with other hospices there are ongoing problems with the timing of referrals. Such a problem is experienced internationally and relates to the curative orientation of doctors (Doyle, 1979:3; Field and James, 1993:13) and the death- denying culture of our society (Pattison, 1977:7). Physicians are seen as the primary gatekeepers of hospice care (Hyman and Bulkin, 1990:39-40). Unfortunately, the majority of physicians do not refer patients, and those that do, refer their patients when they are so close to death that little can be done for them (Siebold, 1992:126).

Referrals are not only one-way. With an acknowledgment of the factor of choice, and a non-judgemental desire to support the wishes of clients, workers from KHS sometimes find the need to refer clients for pain management or in-patient treatment. Consequently, developing contacts of referrals to other palliative care institutions is another aspect of negotiating KHS's existence. As Abel records (1986:78), there are few hospices which can provide the full range of services to the terminally ill in their care. Community hospitals and nursing homes for in-patient care are important services that are needed by community based hospices such as KHS.

World-wide, there is evidence that the hospice concept, which originated as a criticism of mainstream treatment of the terminally ill, has become an accepted part of standard health care. British researchers, such as James and Field (1986:1368), acknowledge the present status of hospice as exemplar players in good practice of terminal care, and influential in policy making. Equally, American authors such as Greer and associates (1986:9) point to the addition of hospice benefits to the Medicare Program (part of the Tax Equity and Fiscal Responsibility Act - TEFRA) as a sign of hospice becoming legitimated as a significant segment of the American health care system. The indications are that hospice has moved from alternative movement to established practice.

There is no such evidence of similar development in Australia, where hospice care and palliation are in the embryonic stage. However, this analysis, situated within the context of hospice literature, suggests that the process of coming into existence of this local service shares much in common with overseas trends.

Conclusion

The theme and focus of this section has been a discussion of the conservative elements in this alternative discourse of the 'exemplary' counterinstitution of the hospice, which has facilitated existence and resistance. Later chapters will take up the argument of how spirituality plays a vital role in KHS's resistance to the biomedical discourse.

Coming into existence, however, is only seen as part of the story when considering issues of resistance and negotiation with mainstream health. As will be outlined in the following chapter, such a process is ongoing, necessitating continuing strategies for survival. The very process of legitimation of KHS by mainstream health, which has so far in the discussion been valued as a factor in ensuring existence, will be shown in later discussions to be a threat to the very organisation it assisted in establishing. There is a 'price' to be paid for support from the hegemonic biomedical system.

Notes

1 When referring to the Australian context, Cheek and Rudge (1993:282) acknowledge that 'the hegemonic discourses of the health system are those of medicine and science.'

2 This mainstream medicocentric powerbase has been referred to as 'medical dominance', by Willis (1989) who writes, 'Two features of the division of labour in health care are immediately apparent. One is its hierarchal nature, the other its domination by one occupation: the medical profession...not only has medicine gained the right to deny the legitimacy of evaluation by others, but it has also gained control over the work of other health organisations' (1989:2-3).

3 The word 'dreaming' as used in this research was coined by participants interviewed and is not suggestive of any link with a similar notion used by Australian indigenous people.

4 As will be elaborated later on in this work, Weber's theoretical understanding is also useful for exploring what Munley refers to as the fourth stage of hospice development: institutionalisation (1983:270). Once a hospice has established itself, gained funding and support from mainstream organisations the process of routinisation challenges the capacity for individual influence and action. As Weber suggest, charisma gives way to routinisation.

5 This perfectionism and overwork in mainstream physicians is well documented covering a broad range of issues from errors made under fatigue conditions, negative experience of internship, emotional impairments and sleep deprivation (Ritchie, 1988:449).

6 The literature not only suggests that staff of hospice projects are seen as highly committed to their work, but, as with KHS contribute to a pool of expertise and source of knowledge which is a resource for others (Clark, 1993:174). As an 'exemplary' organisation their practice is often a model for other organisations. It would be an oversimplification to paint KHS's discourse on the 'people factor' as so unrealistically positive. Throughout the language texts there was ample evidence of self-reflexivity, and an awareness of the ego-needs of individuals. Personality conflicts were a significant tension in this organisation, and at times contributed to

considerable disruption and pain in the life of this service. Such a discussion will be further elaborated on in later chapters of this work. Suffice at present to acknowledge the need to balance the picture.

11 Maintaining existence

This research was undertaken four years after KHS's formation. Not only does this passage of time allow a retrospective examination of this organisation's formation, but also the possibility of exploring the change brought about by stability.

After establishing a service with a spiritual difference, KHS needed to engage in the ongoing process of protecting this difference. This discussion will show that this was (and still is) difficult at best, in a social milieu where the processes of bureaucratisation and professionalisation are arguably inevitable.

Because of the need for funding, referrals and legitimation, KHS is placed in a position of considerable discursive dependence on hegemonic organisations that demand compliance with notions of professionalism and bureaucracy. At a macro-level, resistance is seen to be limited: the power of the system appears to dominate.

However, such ideas about discursive dominance, it will be shown, are an oversimplification of the processes involved. It will be argued that *KHS's spiritual discursive practices play a significant role in deflecting the full power of the system.* An exploration of the notion of spirituality will not only suggest alternative 'ways' of working with the dying whilst maintaining links with the system, but will also begin to challenge the very notion of 'resistance'.

In short the focus of the discussion over the next two chapters is on how KHS, *once it became established, managed to retain its difference in the ongoing struggle against hegemonic processes of professionalism and bureaucratisation.*

The dual purpose of this chapter is: firstly, to articulate the assumptions underpinning *the belief that bureaucratic and professional encroachment on KHS's ideology is inevitable;* and secondly, to demonstrate how, in the face of such 'inevitable power', KHS's discursive response incorporates aspects of *rationalisation 'both/and'*[1] *a Taoist response to such power.*

The next chapter will explore how the notion of spirituality can be seen to be offering some 'freedom' from the demands of such hegemonic power by creating the discursive space for other 'ways' of responding both organisationally and at the coalface when working with the dying. To begin the discussion, however, it is important to introduce some ideas on the notion of resistance.

Resistance is an ongoing process

So far the discussion of KHS's genesis (Chapters 9 and 10) affirms Fairclough's notion (1989:4) that resistance and change is not only possible, but continually happening. A group of 'visionaries', with high ideals and a single minded focus on the goal of hospice formation managed, through dedication, hard work, and the incorporation of the expertise of high profile professionals, to negotiate their existence in a social milieu where there were no similar services.

However, as Fairclough also points out (1989:68), resistance is an ongoing process, as the power 'in' discourse or 'behind' discourse is never permanent, but must be constantly reasserted. Discursive power, which, in the case of KHS, is the opportunity to implement a community based hospice ideology, once won, needs to be exercised and sustained or it will be lost in the course of social struggle between competing interests. Viewed in such terms, the process of coming into being is only part of KHS's story of resistance.

The social reform idea that alternative organisations can challenge the status quo and establish themselves permanently, is viewed here as a linear modernist notion. This postmodern research will focus instead on the ongoing struggle or 'will to power' between mainstream hegemonic organisations and the alternative discourse of this 'exemplary' counter-institution. Coming into existence, it has already been argued, required skills of adaption and compromise to the demands of hegemonic power. Ongoing resistance, to ensure the maintenance of this organisation's survival, also necessitates continual ideological compromise in the face of such hegemonic power, which can be seen to have a demonstrable impact on the discursive practices of the institution.

Consequently, the notion that KHS was able to challenge the status quo and establish itself as a *fait accompli* of social reform will be viewed as a simplistic modernist concept of progress through social change. Within the present postmodern framework, the very factors that assured KHS's successful existence, such as funding, and professionalism, will be problematised as potential ingredients to its own ideological demise.

A return to issues of 'dreaming'

It is important to situate the following comments about organisational change in the context of the hopes and goals of the early members of KHS. As has been expressed by one participant, 'for any change...there has to be a dreaming before there can be a reality' (EQ). For the participants, their discourse on change needs to be understood in terms of the dream they set out to create. *To understand the stress, the 'angst', the ideological challenge created by increasing bureaucratisation and professionalism for KHS, it is important to have a detailed idea of the original vision.* The task for the present discussion becomes one of building up a construction of the complexity of such dreaming.

Such 'dreaming' could simplistically be shown to be based on two important values: firstly, a belief in a democratic, anti-institutional organisational ethos; and secondly, a commitment to holistic patient care. With the vision so stated, an analysis of KHS's resistance could be developed along the dichotomous lines of a unified group of KHS visionaries negotiating their differences with a powerful and opposing discourse. Although attractive because it could be quite easily articulated, such a line of thought has not been chosen for the following two reasons. Firstly, it is not sufficiently sophisticated to reflect adequately the complexity of data collected on this topic. Secondly, such an interpretation would silence the importance of incorporating a multiplicity of voices and ways of seeing, which would negate one of the important reasons for choosing such an approach to this research (as outlined in Chapter 2). Such an interpretative position would prematurely bring closure to understanding and would naively limit both an exploration of the complexity of the dynamic of resistance and an imaginative construction of the many possible directions this organisation could have taken.

Instead, this research acknowledges, explores and affirms the importance of understanding the many voices within the voice of KHS and, by implication, the many alternative possible directions this organisation could have taken. In so doing, this discussion will articulate the creative possibility that, within the discourse of KHS, there could have been (under different circumstances) the construction of quite different 'ways' of responding to the original dreaming. To understand these different possibilities, it is important to start to examine the complexity of the 'talk' on KHS's early dreaming.

The shared vision of a democratic ethos and holistic care

The following language/texts are chosen as examples of the original and the ongoing process of 'dreaming'. They are in addition to those already mentioned in the previous section on this topic and reflect the underlying and continuing anti-bureaucratic ethos.

> So I think that in resisting...hierarchical model people were resisting the dysfunctional things they had seen outside...it won't work here it has not worked anywhere else why should it work here (EQ).

> From day one it has always seemed a challenge I have always seen the need to have this balance between the spiritual side and the professional side, and so always trying to find that balance (EQ).

> He was trying to set up Karuna...as very much in the Buddhist tradition in terms of what it was offering people (EQ).
>
> I see the spirituality...we all have different perspectives and different ways of looking at the truth and I don't think it really matters which perspective we look at it from as long as we have that connectedness that spirituality at the end of it (EQ).

From the beginning, the discursive practices of this organisation were anti-institutional, and anti-bureaucratic: there was a privileging of the spiritual and a desire for human connectedness. The central goal of such anti-institutional dreaming has been described by Punch as,

> an attempt to live perpetually on the margin, resisting the encroachments of formalisation. It is the attempt to retain the spontaneous, immediate, ephemeral joys of 'communitas' against the fate of 'declining' into the norm-governed, institutionalised, abstract nature of law and social structure (1974:312).

The challenge and goal of such discursive practices, according to Punch (1974:313), is the discovery of the secret of continual self-renewal; the avoidance of the rigidity of institutionalisation. Egalitarianism, openness, and flexibility, were the ingredients of the social vision, with liberty and individualism, rather than conformity and collectivism, being the underlying value base (ibid).

Such a vision not only included an anti-institutional orientation for the service organisation, but also an extension of this philosophy to the holistic care of the patient and their family. Such ideas were succinctly expressed by participants as 'a holistic, spiritual approach to death' (EQ) and 'a less institutional way of caring for people' (EQ) which would give patients 'the ability to die where they want and almost how they want' (EQ).

Hospice authors, such as Krant (1974:3), point to the 'world of institutions and technology' that the terminally ill must face, where they experience a loss of control over their world and destiny and become increasingly caught up in the professional and institutional attitudes which inscribes the patient's role as 'combatant to the end'. The KHS dream for patient care evolved from a desire to address such issues.

The shared dreaming for the members of the embryonic Karuna was anti-institutional and anti-bureaucratic, and was founded on a desire to create an alternative, democratic, caring ethos at both the level of organisation and service delivery. As Munley (1983:296) points out, during the early stage of hospice development such focused dreaming is vital, as is the charismatic leadership capable of inspiring the hope and confidence which attracts a committed following, necessary to forge the dream.

The many voices in the shared dream

As the above account of dreaming suggests, KHS's early members were, at least in part, visionaries and idealists. Yet such a description, although a beginning, provides an insufficient account of the early ideological discourse of this organisation, necessary for a discussion on organisational change. *Such unified 'talk' hides the multiplicity of voices and varied constructions of reality possible within such a discourse.*

There are many possible readings of KHS's early vision. Two contradictory but, it will be argued, equally valid constructions will be sanctioned as useful and central to the analysis. The first will be through the eyes of an administrative professional wishing to institute organisational 'reform'. The second, the voice of a professional seeking an alternative way-of-being, or way-of-relating. In many ways, such dichotomous points of view represented the polarity of positions taken during the early formation of this organisation, and hence will form a basis for the following discussion.

KHS's dreaming through the eyes of a professional

The following discussion seeks to show, that individuals associated with the genesis of KHS can be sharing the same vision whilst reading very different and individual ideas into that vision. The first such an individual reading which will be provided is through the eyes of a mainstream health administrator, who came to the fledgling organisation in the hope of making it a professional service. Her vision included the shared dreaming of democratic and holistic goals. However, she saw silenced in that spiritual 'talk' the possibility of 'mismanagement'. With a professional background in health administration, her 'will to power' wanted notions of 'accountability', 'duty of care', and a concern about 'standards' included in such a holistic discourse. As the chief player in KHS's organisational change, this individual 'read' the process of professionalisation and bureaucratisation as 'a growing phase' that was an 'inevitable' evolution to something more desirable. This attitude resonates with Siebold's characterisation (1992:151) of early participants in the hospice movement as 'naive idealists'. Williams amusingly describes them as zealots whose activities resembled,

> ...the old Andy Hardy movies where Mickey Rooney, usually aided by Judy Garland, got the kids of the town mobilised to start a show and raise money for a worthy cause. The first groups to start hospice programs ... were like enthusiastic kids who had little experience or understanding of reality (cited in Siebold, 1992:151).

Although an exaggeration and characterisation, William's description (1990) of the enthusiasm and inexperience of early hospice 'zealots'[2] captures some of the notions silenced in KHS's early discourse. Such visionary talk, although perceived as inspiring at one level, also marginalises important concerns over issues of responsibility and practical experience, which would be challenged by a discourse on professionalism. In the words of the participant recording such concern, 'It wasn't that they didn't care about their clients but they didn't understand that the needs of their clients, they understood a certain part of their client but they didn't understand another part which was sort of that there was always going to be some element of paternalism or maternalism' (EQ). Such a difference in reading the vision was rationalised to the 'frustration of professionals doing business with non-professionals because non-professionals have a very different view of the world' (EQ).

These words privilege the frustration of a professionally oriented individual working in a discourse on care that did not sanction ideas of competence and responsibility as important. For such an individual, KHS's idealistic discursive practices on caring and spirituality, *sous rature*[3] could be exposed to have naive, unrealistic and hence, arguably irresponsible elements. One participant came close to expressing the ideas contained in this understanding, by privileging a negative possibility of the early KHS discourse as,

> Mamby pamby phoney holy wake, you know everybody floating around thinking isn't this wonderful and it is not wonderful. So I would see it go the other way and I had more of a concern in the early days to what we call the cottage industry to me was a bit off with the fairies (EQ).

This first reading of KHS's original dreaming uncovered notions of unrealistic expectations, irresponsibility, lack of professional understanding and expertise, and the possibility of impracticality incapable of achieving the desired ends of excellence in service delivery. Such a reading of KHS's early visionary discourse would argue for incorporating a professional orientation as THE appropriate way of achieving high quality, spiritual care of the dying, and satisfying organisational relationships. This first interpretation of the early dreaming implies a moral imperative to change the service, to incorporate a professional orientation to KHS.

This is the interpretation that has been affirmed by the evolution of this service recorded in the language/texts of this research.

An anti-professional reading of KHS's vision

KHS's original dream could also be placed under erasure in a second way, with implications for a different direction from that which was taken. This second reading of the original goals sanctions, rather than suppresses, the notion of anti-professionalism. The vision is creative; the metaphor is to fashion a pristine object from clay. This reading of KHS's early vision is informed by a desire to serve and a 'will to create': a desire to attain the ideal and utopian circumstances where individuals, both at an organisational and client level, can interact with 'love' and 'compassion'. Such a reading opposes, rather than affirms, the professional bureaucratic notion in mainstream professionalism. The 'will to power' of such an understanding of KHS's original goals would be to resist the encroachment of bureaucratisation, to affirm an evolution into an alternative, counter-institutional form of organisation.

This interpretation of KHS's early discourse is expressed as 'the dream that it could be better, that it could always be pure, that could be real, that it could be more perfect' (EQ). Professionalism is seen in negative terms as the lack of time to care, 'the negative of that (professionalism) which is..we are too busy being professionals to make time to support each other like Buddhists' (EQ).

There was some evidence that such discursive practices did translate into organisational practices which supported an anti-professional ethos (with their arguably irresponsible practices), as demonstrated by the following texts which refer to the early period in KHS's history,

> In the early days, we did the spade work, we did all sorts of things we don't do now. We were not particularly professional, but we had a need to just get up and get referrals, to look after people to start our reputation and so we did things that we wouldn't do now with hindsight (EQ).

However, participants who privileged this second reading of the early dreaming did so with a positive and constructive reference to the importance of *alternative* ways of being caring, loving, compassionate, interconnected human beings. In such a reading, compromise was silenced, and words such as 'pure', 'ideal', and 'perfect' (both in reference to organisational relationships and work with clients) affirmed a profound sense of being alternative to mainstream ways of relating.

Although (as will be demonstrated in the following discussions) KHS did move along the path towards professionalisation (the first reading), this second understanding of KHS's early vision also remained within the organisational 'talk' as a reference point for resistance. *The point is that the shared vision of an organisation based on compassionate, spiritual, holistic care can contain many different interpretative positions about how the end point of that vision can be reached.*

The possibility of many ideological positions

In summary, two quite different interpretations of KHS's original dreaming have been revealed along the professional /anti-professional continuum. It would be an over simplification to argue that such polar opposites were the only positions individuals could take within these discursive practices. Some participants maintain, in fact, that they incorporated both dimensions from the very start, as seen by the following text,

> I said in the very beginning in order to offer a very compassionate service with as many people as possible you have to have a professional and efficient administration and we have to be very professional and organised to offer a compassionate service to people especially as we have grown so much (EQ).

Such a position is seen as a compromise between the polar opposites. The point is that within KHS's one discourse of genesis there were many ideological positions. As Fox (1991:742) explains, postmodern analysis fragments, it offers many new possibilities for understanding action. Rationality is recognised as existing along a continuum of 'rationalities', each reflecting not *truth*, but versions of reality constituted via interests. The path of reason is fragmented to reveal the 'will to power' of the many participants involved in the social practice.

The polar opposites of professionalism/anti-professionalism, or bureaucratic organisation/democratic organisation, will be used as useful constructs for understanding the tension and conflict generated during this part of the organisation's formation. The change in organisational practice and the discursive response to the challenge of such change will be usefully understood by these suggested bipolar opposites.

This discussion has henceforth shown that there were, within the original visionary discourse, many possible ideological positions which could be taken. There were, within the early 'talk' of this organisation, possibilities for several different paths, leading to or away from professionalisation, or a middle path between. Within the one dreaming, it has been shown that there are many possible readings of how that one shared vision can be implemented and understood.

What then was the organisational challenge? What was the new direction that created such ideological angst?

The challenge: a new organisational perspective

> With institutional acceptance came external regulation, standardisation of services, and professionalization (MacDonald, 1990:40).

In the words of the research participant who was seen as responsible for initiating and crystallising the new organisational perspective, the challenge was,

> I brought a new perspective to the organisation that said, yes, we can do this but we also have to be accountable to the people who give us money, we have to be accountable to be with these carers, who expect a certain standard of us and expect us to look after them and we have a duty of care to those people that I took very seriously (EQ).

> I started to standardise everything and I started to say where are our guidelines for things, where are the nursing protocols, where are the protocols for treatments, where are the protocols for how we process patients...if you like where are the by laws of this organisation...where are the administrative and clinical standards, the management standards that you would expect in any specialist organisation anywhere (EQ).

In short, this member sought to bring a professional and bureaucratic administrative standard to the organisation. Such a discourse was not welcomed by the then members of KHS, and strong resistance was demonstrated, as exemplified by the following language/texts,

> People very much wanted to go along with the cottage industry and I wasn't popular because I was challenging that all the time (EQ).

> We don't like those kind of terms. We are quite happy that we have to go along with them, although one or two of them are expressing that they didn't approve, and others were saying we will go along but we will express our concern, and one or two will say I don't like it but I will go with it (EQ).

> My personal concern is why create when you know that this kind of organisational structure that we live in the world isn't very conducive to everybody being satisfied. Why go and create it again? (EQ).

This discussion is concerned with the way KHS responded to such a confrontation with a bureaucratic discourse. KHS was not alone in such a process, as the literature, world wide, suggests that charismatic projects, such as this hospice, once established, move into a period of routinisation and become more bureaucratic in organisational form (James and Field, 1986:1366). Before examining KHS's response in detail, this discussion will be set within the hospice literature which outlines such a recurring process in hospice evolution. Weber's theoretical framework on the evolution from charismatic leadership to bureaucratisation will inform the discussion on this organisational change (Bendix, 1966).

The bureaucratic challenge: understanding the angst

As outlined by Wald and associates (1980:175), the hospice philosophy and ideals to be operationalised, must be situated in the 'real world' of other health care services and funding institutions. For the members of a hospice project to be able to carry out their ideals of care, they must negotiate for funding and approval with health care authorities. It is at this interface between idealists and policy makers that compromise is invited and energies diverted from 'the processes essential in creating an organisation that embodies the founder's principles' (ibid). The present discussion of KHS's ideological challenge sits well within this generic description of hospice evolution.

It is such compromise and diversion that many hospice writers see as the 'threat' to the singleness of purpose which sustained the early hospice movement: the secondary activities, it is argued, are seen to be displacing the primary goal of humane care of the dying (James and Field, 1986:1372). KHS's organisational dilemma is shared by hospices world wide.

One of the most important compromises referred to was that of the increased complexity of hospice organisation. According to Wilkinson and associates

(1990:31), hospices gradually came to resemble the very institutions they sought to replace. Alienation and disillusionment among staff and volunteers was created by this increase in organisational complexity and formality. In short, they record, the 'formal patterns of organisation begin to disrupt informal systems of support and cohesiveness' (ibid). Similarly, the central concern of the members of KHS who resisted such organisational change, focused on the danger the new administrative discourse presented to their 'spiritual way of operating'. The issue from the very beginning (for KHS as well as for hospices worldwide) was a concern to not disrupt the informal systems of support and cohesiveness; above all else to preserve the sense of 'communitas'.

The inevitability of change to bureaucratisation

The nub of the problem thus became, as Punch (1974:312-325) points out, that such a project was 'doomed from the start', as 'communitas' can have no existence independent from the society to which it was a response. This was exacerbated in the case of hospice, where funding and referral depend on negotiating with mainstream bureaucracies. Even without the process of accreditation, the literature indicates that hospices have grown increasingly institutionalised and bureaucratized (Abel, 1986:81). Understandably, the clash between 'visionary' and 'bureaucratic' systems and the differing priorities they purport is recorded as a significant source of collision during hospice development (Clark, 1993:168). This research is but one example of such collision.

The problem of success

So far it has been suggested that as hospices become established, the very ingredients of their success offer a challenge to the ideological singleness of purpose, i.e. humane care of dying people, which sustained the movement in the early stage (James and Field, 1986:1372). The contradiction of success is the threat it contains for ideological destruction. To win is to potentially lose, to succeed is to compromise, to achieve the necessary resources to provide a service is to challenge the very nature of what that service can be. Wald and associates describe such a process in terms of the wider hospice movement, when they state that,

> Hospice practitioners are at risk of being distracted from their original goals by the vast army of professional health workers, consumers, journalists, entrepreneurs, political strategists, management consultants, and fund raisers who, suffused with zeal and a sense of driving mission, have been drawn to the movement..a balance must be struck between the ideals of the reform, on the one hand, and the political and economic realities, on the other..if the ideas are to be kept alive, if a balance is to be

> maintained between ideals and realities, then a tension must develop between the idealists who nourish the ideas and the policy makers who institutionalise them...Yet reformers need credibility, funds, and formal permission to carry out their aims. Decision making inevitably involves compromise, and everyone involved must ask whether the compromise is necessary and, if so, can the ideal survive (1980:173-4).

In short, legitimacy and support from main stream health bring with them demands which impact on the ideological base of hospice organisations.

Once hospice projects have managed to establish themselves, a process known as routinisation is seen to follow (James and Field, 1986). Abel (1986:81) describes the changes during this period to include formalised and sophisticated management structures brought about by funding arrangements, nursing staffs being required to document their services, administrative staff increasingly playing an important role, and the board of the hospice diversifying to include more managerial than the community representation. So distinct is this change that some authors, such as Paradis and Cummings (1986), characterise this process as 'institutional isomorphism'. It is through just a process that hospices become more like each other and similar to other health care settings (Clark, 1993:171).

Such a list of changes resonates with the new administrative direction introduced at KHS during the period of this case study. Guidelines, protocols, and administrative and clinical standards were prepared, nursing staff were forced to attend to administrative tasks such as patient documentation, and business skills were sought from members of the board. The participants recorded the initial impact of such hegemonic demands as 'the most painful period in the organisation's growth', and spoke with concern about their ongoing struggle with such issues. This phase of KHS's evolution thus shares a great similarity to hospice development elsewhere.

An ever increasing aspect of this stage of development is bureaucratisation. As James and Field explain, with routinization comes bureaucracy: 'as the hospices attempted to regularise and stabilise their day to day functioning they became increasingly bureaucratized' (1986:1368).

Such a generic process of hospice evolution is seen as an inevitable move from charismatic movement to routinised bureaucracy. For this reason, as suggested before, Weber's theory of history, which sees social reform, in part, driven by charismatic leadership which later becomes routinised through bureaucracy, will be seen as useful for this discussion.

From charismatic leadership to bureaucratisation

According to the German sociologist Max Weber, reform or change within existing systems begins with dissatisfaction, which is translated through charismatic leadership, among other variables, into a new approach (Kutscher et al., 1983:19). Charismatic leadership, Weber argues from an historical perspective, is often one of the most initially important crystallising and motivating forces for such change. However, when exposed to the pragmatic demands of funding, succession, and service delivery, such charismatic movements inevitably become confronted with the need to create an administrative machine: in short, the process of routinisation begins (James and Field, 1986:1365). According to Weber's interpretation of history, the power and significance of the individual, in this case the charismatic leader, inevitably gives way to 'powers of tradition and rational socialisation' (Bendix, 1966:326). The parallels to KHS's evolution are obvious.

These Weberian notions of the bureaucratisation of charismatic movements can be translated into postmodern understandings of discourse dominance. The bureaucratic challenge of the hegemonic power of mainstream discourse to community based counter institutions, such as KHS, can be understood in Foucaultian terms of power. The Foucaultian notion of power is a relational concept, in which the exponents of one particular discourse (in this case mainstream health professionalism) can limit or direct exponents of a different discourse (in this case a spiritually based hospice organisation) (Cheek and Rudge, 1994:41-2).

Professionalism is described as an inherently conservative discourse, characterised by impersonal rules and procedures laid down by the authorities within the profession (Petersen, 1994:151). Such a conservative discourse is backed by the full discursive power of mainstream biomedical authority. Cheek and Rudge express this idea in Foucaultian terms, stating that, in Western industrial society, 'scientific/medical discourse dominates, often to the exclusion of other types of knowledge, which are dismissed as non-objective, irrational, and unable to be verified by measurement of some kind' (1994:41). The spiritual discourse of KHS is particularly vulnerable to such charges of irrationality and non-verifiable 'truth'.

Hence, in terms of the power/truth nexus, and thus the possibility of ideological praxis, KHS's spiritual discourse would be seen to be particularly vulnerable to being dominated by the hegemonic power of mainstream professionalism and bureaucratic determinism. The power base of KHS's claims to knowledge are situated in marginalised (Buddhism) and alternative (hospice/palliative care) discourses, and hence do not command the 'knowledge power' of mainstream professionalism.

Fairclough, writing from the postmodern understanding of discourse (1989:212), acknowledges the contribution of Weber's ideas on bureacratization and affirms the trend to increasing state control though the expansion of the bureaucratic discourse. Such control or discursive dominance, according to Fairclough, is achieved by the 'colonising' spread of discourse technologies, described as 'types of discourse which involve the more or less self-conscious application of social scientific knowledge for purposes of bureaucratic control. eg. official forms, questionnaires, official records' (1989:213). It was the perceived necessity for introducing such discourse technologies (such as guidelines, protocols, bylaws, management standards) which initiated the 'painful' period of KHS's evolution presently under study. For most of the participants, such a consequentialist, instrumental, bureaucratic rationality was seen to be in direct opposition to the spiritual, democratic, holistic orientation of KHS's original visionaries.

Members of KHS accept the power in the system

So far in this discussion only a theoretical point of view has been presented. It must be stressed, however, that the ruminations of the participants which reflect an ongoing concern and reflection on this issue are not situated in such theoretical knowledge of the inevitability of domination by the system. The view of bureaucratisation and professionalisation, as a *fait accompli* in hospice development, is a theoretical perception, not necessarily shared by the participants. Participants' comments, whilst deferring to the power of the system, entertained the possibility of genuine resistance and pursued the notion of the establishment of alternative practices (this notion will be explored in detail in the next chapter). There was, however, a generalised and stated notion by most of participants as to the lack of choice in future organisational directions, as seen by the following language/texts,

> We realise that at this stage anyway until we find an answer we have to go that way (EQ).
>
> We are going to have to follow more traditional paths of management organisation to make it work comfortably ...even those who are doing it are saying...it doesn't feel right...but I don't see we (have any choice) (EQ).
>
> It had to practically (EQ).

When considering the two (previously outlined) readings of KHS's discourse of genesis, most participants would argue that the first interpretation, which stressed the need to move in the direction professionalism, was inevitable. Certainly, inscribed throughout the language texts is a strong sense that members of this organisation *accepted the move to bureaucratisation in full awareness that they could not offer any other practical solution.*

This does not negate, however, the powerful influence of the idealistic second reading of the original goals and vision. In fact, members of KHS are now even planning a second hospice project which will be built upon different foundations from the present service. Voluntarism and charity will provide the infrastructure for the next service, in place of the government funding and professionalism of the present. Such a service will be an extension of a Buddhist charitable organisation, not a government regional health authority. Consequently, the participants in the new service will be negotiating with quite different discourses, with different interests and investments in their 'will to power'. In the words of one participant, it will be the 'same group of people' but they will 'try and do it all with volunteers and not get the beast of money involved'.

With a different funding infrastructure, or perhaps even a medically trained leader, KHS could have developed in quite different directions. The observations and reflections arising from this research are specific to the many variables which influenced this particular hospice project. As will be discussed in the final chapter on future research agendas, the next KHS project of Cittamini, would provide excellent comparative research material[4] to explore how different social circumstances translate into dissimilarity under the one guiding ideology.

The conclusion of this work, which suggest the inevitability of KHS's present direction towards professionalism and bureacratisation, does not negate the present influence or future possibility of the realisation of the idealistic 'dreaming' in KHS's original vision. In the words of one participant,

> My suspicion is that some people will keep trying, will keep doing that...will keep trying another one... Cittamini or somewhere else and we will see where Cittamini goes...we will follow the dream, I think (EQ).

Summary and recap

So far in this discussion, attention has been drawn to the many different interpretations of KHS's 'dreaming' contained within their shared vision of a democratic organisation that seeks to provide holistic care for the dying. Such a description of the different interpretations of KHS's vision was developed around a professional's view of the visionary discourse as 'naive idealism', as opposed to an idealist's understanding of the vision as an important creative challenge. The tension inherent in this utopian versus professional view of KHS's vision was contextualised to a description and analysis of the challenge of early organisational change experienced by this service. By using Weberian notions of the bureaucratisation of charismatic movements, such change, and the ideological angst it created, was seen to be not only inevitable, but also reflective of a move toward routinisation for hospices world wide. In short, the pragmatic voice of professionalism and bureaucratic management, rather than the visionary voice of the utopian ideal, came to dominate the discourse. This move to bureaucratisation and professionalism was only viewed as inevitable under the circumstances of KHS's need for links with mainstream health for funding, referrals and legitimacy. Under different circumstances, it was suggested that different voices within KHS's dreaming could have come to dominate. One such possibility, for example, is a hospice presently being developed under the auspices of a Buddhist charitable institution which will be run solely by volunteers.

Although the power of the system appears inevitably and increasingly to dominate both KHS and hospice organisations world wide, this is not the complete picture. As the following discussion will show, KHS's spiritual discursive practices were found to play a significant role in protecting the organisation from this full power of the system.

Spirituality: a creative response to the inevitable

The ongoing ideological task thus becomes one of attempting to keep the original spiritual ideals operative, whilst negotiating pragmatic concern of existence situated in the dominant bureaucratic discourse of professionalism. Succinctly stated by one participant, the ideological challenge becomes one of,

> The importance of Karuna having a spiritual base and not turning into a government bureaucracy (EQ).

The hospice literature privileges such a challenge as central to the ongoing survival of hospice ideology and praxis. Solutions offered stress the 'mutual attention between nourishing idealists and the policy makers' (Kutscher et al., 1983:19). Leading authors, whilst accepting the need for the new wave of professional managers, stress the imperative role of idealists as essential to keeping alive the original dream, and to preventing the hospice alternative from 'falling into the rigid patterns of bureaucracy' (Munley, 1983:296).

Exploring idealism: an important outcome of this research

This whole notion of the role and importance of idealism, which translates into KHS's spiritual discourse, is considered to be of central significance in this research.

The following discussion (which includes chapter 12) will explore this interface between a spiritual discourse and the power inherent in the hegemonic professional and bureaucratic discourses. In line with the postmodern theoretical framework, comments will be restricted to the insights arising directly from the statements of participants. Comments will be ad hoc, local and contextual. Such a spiritual discourse will be shown to have multiple and often contradictory effects.

Firstly, the powerlessness in such a spiritual discourse will be explored, with a suggestion that such 'talk' is, to some degree, a rationalisation based on conservative notions of acceptance of the inevitable power of the system. The spiritual idealism, which contributed so strongly to the genesis of the organisation, it will be proposed, converts to rationalism in the face of the awesome power of the system. This is however, only part of the story.

Secondly, the Eastern spiritual dynamic in this discourse will be sanctioned as a positive possibility for effectively relating to the power within the system. Such a dynamic will be seen to resemble a Tao of power, an ability to flex in the face of insurmountable difficulties: in short, a spiritual dynamic that contributes to creating a difference, not by opposition but by effectively 'going with the flow'.

In the next chapter, it will be argued that such a spiritual discourse can also provide the discursive space and a subjectivity which can deflect, quite substantially, the dehumanising influence of mainstream ways of seeing. This will be shown to be operating at both the organisational level and at the coalface of work with families. Such a different way of 'speaking the world' translates into different organisational relationships and different 'ways' of working with the terminally ill.

In summary, KHS's spiritual discourse will be shown to be not only a most important determining factor in the genesis of this service, but also an ongoing influence on the maintenance of its difference. The conclusion is, that, in the light of such an understanding, KHS's spiritual dynamic can be seen as *the* connecting ingredient that underpins and sustains the different 'way' this organisation works with the dying.

As no discourse is exempt from its own particular 'will to power', the spiritual discourse of KHS will also be uncovered to reveal the possibility of coercive, and arguably unethical, possibilities in its application (Chapter 12).

A beginning will be to explore the notion of spiritual rationalisation.

Introducing notions of spiritual rationalism

Fairclough, defines rationalisation as explanations,

> which cannot be taken at face value but are themselves in need of explanation ... rationalisations as part and parcel of naturalisation: together with the generation of common-sense discourse practices comes the generation of common-sense rationalisations of such practices, which serve to legitimise them (1989:92).

The process of naturalisation, in relation to the present discussion of KHS, refers to the acceptance of professionalisation and bureaucratisation as 'common sense' within this service. Certainly, the person seen as chiefly responsible for organisational change brought with her such a notion that her new perspective was 'common sense', inevitable, proper, and legitimate, as can be seen by her comment that, 'it is not a death, it is a just a new growing phase that the organisation goes through and you might have a complete turn over of people in that process, but that is the nature of organisational change' (EQ). For this organisational member, such change 'was an inevitable thing that had to happen' (EQ).

Although such practices were eventually seen as inevitable, or unable to be resisted and hence naturalised, this was only a partial process for two reasons. Firstly (as outlined in the previous discussion on the differing readings of KHS's original dreaming), not all members of KHS accepted the direction towards new organisational change. Some who were very opposed to the direction left the organisation. Others, whilst staying and agreeing to such change, did so with reluctance and a sense of a lack of another alternative. Some, it must be added, neither questioned nor disapproved of the new perspective. There was, in short, heterogeneity in the discursive practices of legitimation and naturalisation.

Secondly, there was, and still is, a considerable conscious awareness of these issues within the every day talk of this organisation. To explore this issue fully it is again necessary to return to definitions. Fairclough defines naturalisation as follows,

> ...if a discourse type so dominates an institution that dominated types are more or less entirely suppressed or contained, then it will cease to be seen as arbitrary (in the sense of being one among several possible ways of 'seeing' things) and will come to be seen as natural, and legitimate because it is simply *the* way of conducting oneself. I will refer to this, as the naturalisation of a discourse type...naturalisation is the royal road to common sense (1989:91).

Although it can be confidently argued that the practice of professionalism and bureaucratisation dominates the organisation of KHS, it would be very difficult to state that there is an ideological homogeneity around these practices, or that they had been naturalised. This dominant discourse, so to speak, has not entirely suppressed nor contained other ways of seeing. The new organisational perspective is accepted to a degree as inevitable and 'common sense' in a competitive world of health professionalism, but it is not ideologically affirmed by all members of the service as a positive and desirable direction. In short, the new direction in organisational management has not been naturalised to ideological common sense.

This heterogeneity of discursive practices on organisational management, and conscious awareness of the impact of the new organisational direction on the spiritual discourse, are, it is argued, key ingredients when considering this example of KHS's experience with power struggles for control over discourse types. The point is that neither the social determination, nor effect of the discourse types are 'hidden' and 'indirect' from the members of KHS. In short, the 'opacity of discourse' (Fairclough, 1989:41), an important ingredient in legitimation and sustaining of power through discourse, is not operating as a factor in KHS. The members of KHS are very aware of both the 'power behind the discourse(s)' (professionalism/bureaucratisation), and their ideological desire to resist such discursive dominance. The need for consciousness raising, usually viewed as a preliminary act towards liberation from the dominance of powerful discourse types (Fairclough, 1989:41; 1992:12), is not necessary in this context. There already exists a consciously conceived and clearly articulated oppositional stance by many members of this organisation to the encroachment of a professional and bureaucratic discourse.

As an extension of the above inscribed ideas, it is argued that, although professionalism and bureaucratisation have come to dominate the practices of KHS, there has not been a parallel discursive process of naturalisation. The spiritual discourse of KHS has remained consciously articulated and ideologically resistant to the intrusion of such practices.

Beginning to ask questions

In the face of such power within the system are the participants' comments that indicate a spiritual resistance perhaps a form of rationalisation by individuals who feel suppressed or contained by hegemonic power? Or is there, instead, a substantive rationality in the spiritual discourse which may offer some hope of the possibility of ongoing resistance? As stated in the introduction to this chapter, the argument that such discursive practices reflect both rationalisation and the creation of a discursive space for resistance will be developed. Notions of spirituality can both protect and inspire; such ideas can give the illusion of choice in a situation of powerlessness whilst, at the same time, creating an ideological space for difference in action. This effect will be shown to vary, being less likely to operate with success at the organisational level, and more likely at the interface between service and client. A marginalised discourse at the macro (or organisational) level may only offer minimal resistance, but could arguably be a powerful point of resistance at the micro-level of the individual (ideas discussed in full in Chapter 12).

Spirituality, rationalisation and the organisational dimension

In keeping with the notion of the heterogeneity of KHS's discursive practices on this issue, it is important to note that rationalisation of professionalism will depend on the perspective of the speaker. Some members of KHS rationalised, without opposition, a positive notion of bureaucratic management and professionalisation, as demonstrated by the following language/text,

> There still has to be some degree of hierarchy if for no other reason than to support people at the bottom of the hierarchy there has to be someone for them to pass the buck to (EQ).

Even for those who did not believe in the direction of change, there was evidence privileging a positive notion of the outcome and hence justifying such change. The Utilitarian ethical concept of the greatest good for the greatest number was the *raison d'etre* of such rationalisation in the face of unwelcome change. The following language/texts privilege such notions,

> The bottom line has to be that more people die at home today than they did three years ago...and that in itself justifies it (EQ).

> It is the funding that has allowed us to greatly improve our service (EQ).

Such statements are paradigmatic examples of rationalisations, which privileged a pragmatic but positive notion of the importance of accepting the demands of the system so as to be able to implement KHS's practical ideals. These were the most common rationalisation. The motivation behind such rationalisation was the need to positively frame the belief that there were few other options, as seen by the following statements,

> I don't think anyone set out to use terms that negotiated with mainstream

> but we recognised the fact that if we were going to get funding we had to use the right jargon (EQ).

> I mean what does it matter what someone is called, what does it matter...so I think people saw no harm in just using the name and the shell within the structure...because I mean it is us who is doing it (EQ).

When members of KHS were forced, by mainstream health, to use position names and organisational patterns that were counter to their democratic and holistic spiritual goals, there was a readiness to use rationalistic statements of justification. At the organisational level, such rationalisation can also be translated as flexibility and the capacity to 'fit in'. While this can be seen as a process of rationalization and conformity, it can also be seen in a very different way, and one which speaks of a different relationship to power than linear Western notions of resistance or opposition. These ideas will now be explored.

Karuna's Tao of power

> 'By gentle and skilful means based on reason' - From the Mongolian Buddhist Tradition (Paige and Gilliatt, 1991).

When talking about resisting the hegemonic power of the system, participants did not use words such as opposing, attacking or fighting the system. They spoke rather of notions of fitting in, of 'going with the flow', with the aim in mind of achieving their spiritual goals of service to the community, as can be seen by the following extract,

> We have got to make it work with what is here not make it so impossible that it would do nothing... Karuna has tried to fit in...if it says the government has rules, if it says there are job descriptions, if it says there are fund raising, it acknowledges the very framework we have to work in rather than trying to create something that is not in this real..you know..it is a nice little cottage industry up in the hippy mountains somewhere you know...I don't see that as being a benefit to anybody (EQ).

There was an articulated and conscious awareness that the way to achieve spiritual aims of working holistically with the dying was through co-adaptation, not opposition, to the system. In the words of one participant, the challenge in relating to issues of power and change is to adapt or 'die': 'because it has to transform, it has to change. You can't make the things around it change to fit it' (EQ).

Indeed, the members of KHS were 'successful' in implementing their goals. Any consideration of the spiritual discourse, must then take this success into consideration. Far from just a rationalisation of the enormous power of the system, KHS's spiritual discourse also contains a transformative power, which means that a small group of visionaries were able to eventually establish a service against what has already been described as considerable odds. As has already been outlined, although achieved with the help and legitimation of the system, such a service has maintained its difference with regards to important issues, such as a caring, holistic, twenty four hour service, the provision of choice, and the opportunity to die at home.

According to participants, KHS's success came through its ability to 'merge with' and validate the system, as seen by the following comment which contrasts it with the home birth movement,

> I think that is where the home birth movement eventually failed. They attracted an airy fairy high fluting people so that they could never actually infiltrate into the hospital medical system and they are still even now having to come to terms with that because they really had an attitude of invalidation of the system rather than emerging with it and trying to work within it whereas I feel Karuna has done that (EQ).

In view of such comments, the notion of resistance used in this research needs to be changed. A move from the more oppositional and perhaps antagonistic flavour, to one of achieving ends and making a difference through working with hegemonic influences is suggested. Such a notion resembles a Taoist understanding of power, as summed up by Page, when he writes,

> The way out of our uneasiness is to observe change, and to flow intelligently with it. This is *wu wei,* a process which can be likened to the skilful way in which a yachtsman uses the wind and the tide (both at times contrary) in order to reach port (1989:60).

The Taoist challenge is to 'look out for the grain of things and work with it and things are made simpler' (Watts, 1971). Such an Eastern Taoist notion is compatible with KHS's spiritual discourse, which is underpinned by Buddhist beliefs. Buddhist teachings emphasise, as has been outlined previously, that the ingredient for change comes from within the individual. For the Buddhist, antagonistic and conflictual relationships are to be avoided. Through a deep understanding of the doctrine of the no-self, a balanced and serene attitude is cultivated in relating to others (Chau, 1991:94).

For the Buddhist,

> Better it is to conquer oneself
> Than to conquer others,
> None can undo the victory
> Of one who is self-mastered
> And always acts with self-restraint,
> Though one conquers in battle
> A thousand times a thousand men,
> Yet the greatest conqueror is
> One who conquers self
> (Dhammapada 104-103 cited in Ross, 1994).

As outlined in a previous chapter on Buddhism, the orientation of this Eastern philosophy towards problems in the social world is not to focus on altering the outside environment, but rather to cultivate an individual spirituality. Indeed, the fourth noble truth of Buddhism is the path of self-transformation (the dharma): an eightfold path advocating right belief, right thought, right speech, right conduct, right livelihood, right endeavour, right awareness, right meditation (Ross, 1993:161). According to Buddhist philosophy, there is an element of existential choice, even in oppressive situations. How the individual workers of KHS interact with others at an organisational level, according to this philosophy, depends as much on a spiritual orientation as any external circumstances. Spiritual choice can consequently be translated into 'right action'. Compassion and wisdom can be exercised no matter what the sociological conditions. Such an idea has been expressed succinctly in the following language text,

> Rather than change what is going on outside, you change what is going on in yourself, so that is true Buddhism (EQ).

Understandably, then, such a discourse endorses accommodation and co-adaption to the system.[5] This notion of flexing in the face of power and change in an attempt to protect and nurture the growth of the embryonic KHS resonates throughout the language/texts. This idea of 'going with the flow', rather than relying on resisting, confronting or proselytising, it will be argued, is an Eastern notion of spiritual praxis which is essential for understanding a very positive aspect of KHS's spiritual discourse.[6]

Conclusion

This research affirms, and contribute a concrete example of the theoretical observation that spirituality, although a most important ingredient in the discourse of genesis of community based hospices, in the long term, can convert to rationalisation at the macro-level of organisational practice. A spiritual discourse is the usual prerequisite for the initiation and implementation of a hospice project. The vision, commitment and dedication needed to sustain such a project in the initial stages are expressions of the spiritual motivation. Such a spiritual dimension, however, does not, according to the findings of this research, offer any substantial protection to the implementation of a democratic, and alternative practice once the service is established. Spiritual rationalisation, not resistance, is the likely outcome at an organisational level, once the service begins to negotiate with mainstream organisations.

However, the spiritual dynamic of KHS is more complex than this notion of rationalisation, as the discussion has shown. Within the Buddhist based spiritual discourse of KHS was a flexible relationship to power, which challenged the notion of resistance used so far in this research. Such a relationship to power was expressed in terms of a Taoist understanding of the importance of 'going with the flow'.

The spiritual discourse of KHS was thus shown to contain elements of rationalisation 'both/and' alternative ways of responding to power. As this is only part of the interpretation that was developed, the discussion which follows will further elaborate on Karuna's spiritual discourse, taking into consideration the important notions behind its successful implementation of a service with a difference.

Notes

1 'Both/and' is a Derridian term (Lather, 1991:105) coined to replace the modernist binary logic of 'either/or'. As Bauman suggests (1993:5), 'the point is precisely that modern life does not abide by the "either/or" of logic.' In the present context this term refers to the contradiction of a spiritual discourse engaged at the same time in a powerless and a powerful relationship to a hegemonic discourse: the spiritual discourse is the vehicle for accepting powerlessness as well as a powerful means to gain the organisation's desired ends. As Bauman points out, 'contrary to logic, this does not necessarily mean that one of the accounts is false' (ibid), for even where 'there is a logical contradiction between two accounts' postmodern notions of deconstruction allows the interpretation to move beyond the limits of binary logic. This conceptual freedom to hold two contradictory notions at the one time is valued in this research.

2 Such an interpretation of KHS's early discourse, will be interpreted as too harsh. Particularly, if taking into account, the already outlined consciously conceived process of the creative incorporation of resources such as individuals with expertise, knowledge, prestige and the hard work and dedication of the early members of this service. However, such a description does inscribe the 'naive idealist' notion that is useful for the present discussion.

3 The term 'sous rature' was first coined by Derrida and literally translated means 'under erasure' which refers to the process of deconstruction as outlined in Chapter 2. According to Atkins (1983:17), 'he writes a word, crosses it out, and prints both word and deletion, for though the word is inaccurate it is necessary and must remain legible. This idea of 'sous rature' is an analogue of the undoing/preserving play that everywhere characterises, indeed creates, Derridean thought'.

4 Indeed, researchers in health such as Willis (1994:5) call for an exercising of the social imagination through an exploration of such structural issues as a prerequisite for developing the critical sensitivity necessary for the search for more satisfactory alternative futures in health care.

5 Buddhists are noted for their remarkable ability to adapt to local conditions. Ch'en (1968:268) notes that 'In every land where Buddhism has been introduced, the religion has displayed remarkable elasticity in adapting itself to local conditions and in responding to new needs. Probably no other missionary religion has this characteristic to such a remarkable degree.'

6 Understandably, Buddhists support and advocate nonviolent global problem-solving (Paige and Gilliatt, 1991).

12 Spirituality: making the difference

> In Foucault's view, there is an inextricable link between knowledge and power. However, he rejected the idea that power is a system of domination that controls everything and that leaves no room for freedom. He argued that wherever power relations operate there is always resistance. Power does not operate directly on the individual to control him or her, but rather serves to guide the conduct of individuals and groups in institutions, and there is always some *freedom* (Petersen, 1994:7).

In continuing to develop the notion of the impact of KHS's spiritual discourse on the struggle against mainstream bureaucratisation and professionalisation, this discussion will now focus on the above mentioned Foucaultian notion of 'freedom'. The notion of 'freedom' refers in this case, to the process by which KHS is able to maintain its vision and values in spite of the pressures from external organisations. The idea that 'there is always some freedom' to resist will be forwarded to counterbalance the theorising in the previous chapter, which pointed to the inevitability of KHS's domination by the hegemonic discourse of biomedicine. Such 'freedom' will be described in terms of KHS's spiritual discourse, the argument being, that *the 'talk' of this organisation provides the discursive space* [1] *and a subjectivity which creates, supports, and attracts spiritual ways of seeing and acting which can offer some resistance to the dehumanising aspects of biomedicine's demands.*

By responding constructively to the system's demands, KHS has gone a long way to meeting its own spiritual goals, but at the same time expresses an ongoing angst about the 'price' of such a compromise. These concerns and tensions faced by KHS in their ideological struggles are central to the spiritual apprehension voiced in the literature surrounding the present hospice experience throughout the world. In the words of Wald and associates,

> The hospice movement is at the threshold of acceptance by government

and the medical establishment. Of immediate consequence, therefore, is the way the movement shifts from a peripheral and reform role to integration within the health care system. The task ahead is to maintain values and standards while allowing innovation, accepting regulation, and adapting to existing structures (1980:178).

The following discussion will attempt *to make a contribution to understanding this issue,* which is considered of central importance to hospices world wide. In keeping with the postmodern tenets already outlined, such a contribution is ad hoc, contextual and local. The story is of the response of one hospice to such issues.

Central to this understanding is the notion that spiritual beliefs can offer some resistance to the dehumanising aspects of professionalisation and bureaucratisation. The language/texts certainly privilege the notion of a 'gentle spirituality' being a positive contribution and operational factor in the organisational life of KHS.

This spiritual dynamic will be explored at the level of organisational relationships and at the coal face of patient care. At both these levels, the 'discursive magnet' will be interpreted as an important factor reinforcing this organisation's efforts of resistance. The discourse magnet (Chapter 10) is a process which attracts to this organisation like-minded individuals who are appreciative of the spiritual vision. In contrast to this, negative factors such as the pain, hurt, and grief resulting from personality conflicts and the possible unethical use of this spiritual discourse will be introduced as possible blocks to spiritual resistance.

At the coalface of patient care, the spiritual praxis will be construed as being of considerable consequence as a process protecting and maintaining this organisation's vision and values. KHS's spiritual discourse, it will be argued, creates and supports both a caring worker subjectivity and a holistic perception of the patient and his/her family's needs. Such processes, translated into patient care, will be interpreted as key factors contributing to this organisation's resistance to the dehumanising processes of biomedicine's response to death and dying. By implication, such factors will be linked to the innumerable positive reports on this organisation's work, which was the initial reason for beginning this research (as outlined in Chapter 1 and Chapter 3).

In summary, then, it will be suggested that, KHS's psycho-spiritual discourse although easily dominated by hegemonic notions of professionalism and bureaucracy, can when translated into a particular form of subjectivity, arguably be seen as a point of some resistance. This resistance operates both at the organisational level and at the coalface of patient care. Such an argument needs to be situated within a postmodern understanding of subjectivity.

Introducing the notion of subjectivity

According to Davies (1994:23), discourses create the possibilities for certain subject positions through which the individual interacts with others. Part of the effect of discursive practices is shaping or actualising certain ways of being, of speaking about the world, and hence, is constitutive of the persons who adopt them (Davies, 1994:44). The individual, as 'author' of statements, cannot be viewed as an entity outside of, and independent to, discourse, but is rather a function, or effect, of the discourse itself (Fairclough, 1992:43). There is a direct and creative link between discourse and the subjectivity of the individual. Fairclough (1992:45) would advocate that such a creative link is a dialectical one, with subjectivity being shaped by discursive practices, but also able to have an influence on reshaping and restructuring such practices.

As Fairclough outlines (1989:39), although social subjects are constrained to operate, somewhat passively, in the subject positions set up in discourse types, they can also act as active and creative social agents. Importantly for this discussion, Fairclough clearly states,

> Subjects are ideologically positioned, but they are also capable of acting creatively to make their own connections between the diverse practices and ideologies to which they are exposed, and to restructure positioning practices and structures. The balance between the subject as ideological 'effect' and the subject as active agent, is a variable which depends upon social conditions such as the relative stability of relations of domination (Fairclough, 1992:91).

Even within a wider context of discursive domination, the individuals within KHS, can operate as agents of resistance and change, asserting their spiritual ideology on a micro-basis.

It will be a central tenet of the argument developed that, although the awesome power of domination and surveillance as understood in Foucaultian notions of knowledge/power is acknowledged, there is some discursive space, in a community based hospice organisation such as KHS, to exercise a degree of meaningful ideological resistance at the level of the individual or, in postmodern term, the 'active agent'. Such resistance can be seen to be translated into both organisational structure and client service.

Creating the spiritual space, not changing the system

> To provide the space you at least have to have an idea of that spiritual self (EQ).

At the micro-level, the notion has been introduced that individuals can participate as active agents with creative potential in developing connections between ideology and practice (Fairclough, 1992:91). In this discussion, the idea of the active agent, is not particularly concerned with the concept of the dialectical relationship between discourse and social structure (Fairclough, 1989:37). It is acknowledged, however, that KHS's discourse on spirituality has the creative potential, especially through the process of public education and provision of an effective alternative choice in terminal care, to make an impact on the very discourse which it seeks to replace. Although a dialectic may very well exist between the mainstream biomedical discourse and the 'exemplary' practices of KHS, this is not the present focus of discussion.

The resistance of the active agent referred to here is more concerned with *the creation of a spiritual space whereby the individual,* ***in spite of*** *the demands from more powerful discourses, can* ***choose*** *to act with difference.* This notion that the individual's commitment to a spiritual way of seeing can act as a protection to dehumanising practices is clearly expressed in the words of the participants' as follows,

> I think that there are some exceptionally wonderful people in operating in Karuna and they will do their best to maintain that special stuff (EQ).
>
> There are some people in there who are spiritual to the core and as long as they are there they will keep it (EQ).
>
> If we hang on to those kind of people we will survive and we will keep our spiritual way of doing it (EQ).
>
> All of us were coming from a very spiritual base, spirituality, sort of, you know, influenced us (EQ).

The subjectivity supported by the expression of KHS's spiritual discourse includes notions of compassion, gentleness, and a willingness to serve and strive for excellence. A summary of the key attitudinal ingredients of KHS's discourse on spirituality as expressed by participants in this research incorporates,

- a desire to serve
- a tolerance of multiplicity in thought and action
- self actualisation through interconnectedness and altruism
- compassion inscribed as love and caring kindness
- selfless or 'pure' motivation
- integration of spiritual practices in everyday life
- holistic care of the individual
- life as a spiritual journey

A subjectivity informed by such a way of 'speaking the world' would, understandably, be attractive to, and supportive of, individuals who sanction a loving, caring and gentle way of relating to each other and the families with which they work. Equally, such a discourse is likely to marginalise more ego centric, aggressive ways of being. Throughout the interviews, such a disapproval of hostile or pushy actions did surface as examples of individuals who were seen as 'not coming from a gentle spiritual base' (EQ). 'A gentle way of doing things'(EQ) was voiced as an important quality needed in members of this organisation, particularly as the service expands.

By outlining KHS's expressed subjectivity as gentle does not necessitate, *ipso facto*, that this organisation only attracted individuals with a peaceful and sensitive way of relating. The language/texts provide considerable detail of conflictual personality dynamics. Such times of conflict, however, were described as 'incredibly painful periods' of this service's evolution and contrasted to the present 'espirite de corpes' which has been described as 'never been better'.

The point is thus that *KHS's spiritual discourse shapes a subjectivity, which attracts and supports individuals who are comfortable with a gentle, caring, tolerant, and dedicated way of seeing the world*: a way of seeing that includes an understanding of the centrality of meaning making. Such a subjectivity contrasts with the notions outlined in the biomedical system (Chapter 7).[2]

A return to the bio-medical model

To understand the full significance of KHS's spiritual subjectivity, it is important to contrast it with the corresponding subjectivity of the biomedical model. This discussion, it is important to note, is concerned with the subjectivity created by biomedicine, not the individual qualities of practitioners within such a system. Although qualities of caring and compassion are generic throughout the health care system, different discourses, it will be argued, either restrict or foster the expression of such qualities. The same health professionals can find themselves acting very differently in dissimilar discourses.

As outlined in Chapter 7, mainstream medicine is guided by an engineering approach to the body, professionals are perceived as biotechnicians, and profit, income and status are motivating forces in such physical care (Ratcliff, 1989:173). In contrast to the gentle, holistic subjectivity of KHS, the scientific, mechanistic biomedical model is predicated on notions of medicocentrism, which rewards its players with power and privilege (Freund and McGuire, 1991). Such medical dominance is maintained by expert control through specialised knowledge about the body, which excludes, or makes subservient, other workers and the patient (Armstrong, 1987:1214). As Fisher outlines this position,

> Doctors who are oriented almost exclusively to the technical bioscientific aspects of medicine have the dominant voice. They speak in the voice of medicine while patients who are subordinate have difficulty inserting the voice of the lifeworld, have difficulty getting heard (1991:159).

Medicocentric control and dominance underpins the subjectivity of mainstream health discourse. This was expressed clearly by one of the participants when she stated simply,

> Nurses are inclined to be a bit bossy anyway and the medical profession is inclined to be in control (EQ).

Subjectivities with a difference

To reiterate, the present discussion is predicated on the notion that discursive practices are constitutive and formative of social subjectivity. In the words of Weedon, discourses are,

> ...more than ways of thinking and producing meaning. They constitute the 'nature' of the body, unconscious and conscious mind and emotional life of the subjects which they seek to govern. Neither the body nor thoughts and feelings have meaning outside their discursive articulations, but the ways in which discourse constitutes the minds and bodies of individuals is always part of a wider network of power relations, often with institutional bases (1987:108).

Subjectivity, so interpreted, is different from the earlier Western psychological concept of identity, which privileges a notion of the unitary, non-contradictory self (Davies, 1994:3). Individual subjectivity, according to this interpretation, is context-dependent, positioned and constituted by discourse and hence power relations (ibid).

Using this notion of subjectivity (as context dependent and constituted by discourse), committed, dedicated, altruistic health professionals would have different opportunities available to them for expressing their caring, depending on whether they were in a biomedical or spiritual discourse. The same individual would feel support for very different actions in different discourses. This notion was expressed by a participant when he stated,

> The compassionate nurse at the hospital is extraordinarily busy and doesn't have the time to sit down and hold the patient's hand and talk with them about it. That is the difference. They don't have the resources like volunteers to offer the same degree of care that we give, because we place more emphasis if you like on the emotional and spiritual aspects of care. It is just the numbers. They don't have time. They would if they could (EQ).

It must be understood that it was not the individual worker's caring, *per se,* which was the significant factor in determining holistic and compassionate care of the dying, but rather the support for interpreting and expressing such altruistic behaviour which is available within an organisational discourse. One participant made reference to this point when talking about 'caring and compassionate' physicians who are attracted to KHS's 'spiritual environment'. This participant stated,

> ...because they are all very caring and compassionate people...that is the key ingredient and I don't think that is unique; and I think all you could say is that Karuna has a concentration of those sort of people...the medical system they are all through, and they come here and get drawn to Karuna because they see that perhaps the environment that they are working in, is perhaps not as strong as they would like it to be, and so want to come here

where they can see it more concentrated and they can work more in a spiritual environment. But they come here because already they have those qualities (EQ).

Consequently, this notion of subjectivity has important implications if understood in terms of the discourses running through KHS. Whilst it is acknowledged that the members of this organisation did significantly defer in their discursive practices to the hegemonic notions of mainstream health, this has only been part of the story. The very fact that a spiritual discourse is privileged in the language/texts and is valued, and not marginalised, by this organisation suggests, *ipso facto,* that some discursive space exists for a spiritually informed subjectivity.

Such a dynamic can only be understood in terms of the all embracing significance of the spiritual discourse within this organisation. As has already been outlined in the discussion on rationalisation, such discursive practices can be, and are, maintained in the face of serious compromise to the demands of mainstream health. In the face of significant and obvious concessions to more dominant discourses, the members of this service still comfortably privilege the possibility and value of a 'gentle spirituality'.

So privileged is this discourse within KHS that members speak of themselves in descriptions reflective of valued spiritual characteristics. Examples from the language/texts include,

> Proudly I could say that I was very caring for individuals and other human beings and respecting people's rights to do it their way (EQ).
>
> (What) we are looking for is a person, not who is a perfect person or a saint, but who is a genuinely compassionate person...people who can express their warmth, their love, their compassion and their willingness to serve others (EQ).
>
> (We attract people)...who actually live what they believe and I think Karuna is made up of people who are living out what they believe (EQ).
>
> There is some very special, some very loving feelings that happen everyday in that place (EQ).
>
> ...so what is unique about it is the people who are involved in it and their constructive energy (EQ).

Such a subjectivity, privileges, supports and reinforces the possibility of spiritually inscribed ways of seeing and acting. As already outlined (Chapter 4), KHS's spiritual subjectivity was considered to be a significant factor contributing to their expressed difference.

This way of seeing, and way of being, contrasts greatly with the already outlined discourse on mainstream medicine. *Different discourses, it is argued, translate into different subjectivities: different ways of seeing and valuing the self as worker and colleague.*

In summary, it has been argued that a discursive space exists in the discourses running through KHS for a spiritually inscribed subjectivity. Such a subjectivity, it is suggested, offers the possibility of existential choice, 'speaking the world' (Davies, 1944:44), of existing, which may be suppressed or at best marginalised in biomedical organisational settings. A subjectivity based on 'compassion', 'love', and 'caring', it is argued, would go some way to building-in resistance to the depersonalising elements in the discourse of professionalism and bureaucratisation.

Participants certainly privilege, as possible and essential, such practices of resistance, as seen by the following language/texts,

> We would value that space and still see that space as a very powerful thing (EQ).

> They might talk about being positive or being healthy or giving another label, but what they are actually talking about is their spiritual selves, what the Christians call the holy spirit, what the Buddhist's call the pure essence, that aspect of them that can really change things and I think that is what makes Karuna unique (EQ).

> (We) just have to have patience to one another and their ideas..and that is what we are hanging on to (EQ).

Taking into account the discursive magnet

It would be too simplistic to suggest that KHS's spiritual discourse can be understood as a one way process of creating a humanising space for members of this organisation to express, and be supported in, their caring attitudes to others. The discursive dynamic is more complex than this. There is an active ingredient expressed in the talk about the players who fill the discursive space. Participants use words such as 'we are looking for' or 'filtering people with a gentle spirituality' suggesting an operative link with individuals outside the organisation.

As has been previously outlined, KHS has a discourse that attracts others of similar mindedness. Likened to a discursive magnet, the spiritual talk at KHS is seen to 'vibrate' and 'hook certain people'. This dynamic is explained as a process 'kind of like preaching to the converted' in which 'Karuna attracts certain people'. There is, in short, both an attraction and 'filtering' of people who eventually become involved in KHS's discursive practices.

Viewed in terms of such a dynamic, KHS's discourse is seen not only to create a discursive space sympathetic to achieving its goals, but also to attract the very people suitable to, and sympathetic with, such discursive practices. In short, the discourse creates, supports, and attracts. Energy is not expended in changing, proselytising and convincing.

The link between spiritual praxis and personality dynamics

This is not to argue that, because this service has created a positive spirituality which attracts likeminded individuals and supports them in their efforts to care for others, the experience will be invariably positive and constructive.

The language/text, whilst privileging the idea of constructive and nourishing relationships built on a notion of spiritual caring, also inscribes the pain, hurt, and grief of individual experiences with this service. As with any organisation and, indeed, similar to a comparable hospice service in Geelong, KHS experienced serious problems of conflict and fallout, of power politics, sexist relationships and personality clashes. Key figures who worked with dedication and commitment left with grief and hurt, cutting contact with the organisation, often both formal and informal. Some indication of the depth and breath of this phenomena can be sampled from the following comments by participants,

> Change is inevitable..the only thing I see as a problem is the personality clashes (EQ).

> I think of the times obviously when personal dynamics come into it, people take sides ... team not working the fallout is enormous (EQ).

> It was an incredibly painful period in our growth (EQ).

> I think what made it very difficult were personality issues (EQ).

> It really brought on a personal crisis (EQ).

> There was male and female stuff, there was control and power, this was real sexism at work..carefully disguised but basically deadly sexist stuff..about straight power (EQ).

> ...it is to do with personalities (EQ).

> It is very much a male driven organisation (EQ).

> I feel there is a sadness, I feel sad that people were hurt because there were a lot of people got hurt (EQ).

A balance to such statements is the assessment by participants that the present 'esprit de corps' of KHS has never been better.

The important point here is that, just because an organisation affirms a spiritual perspective and is successful in creating and supporting a discursive space and subjectivity which expresses a spiritual way of seeing and acting, this does not *ipso facto* imply that it will necessarily be free of the potentially destructive aspects of personality conflicts. KHS's spiritual discourse, it has been argued, makes an important contribution to, but is not necessarily an absolute protection of, caring, harmonious organisational relationships.

Such a statement would be the starting premise for further research, not a conclusive statement for this research. The language/texts suggest further questions rather than any definitive conclusion on the topic (such questions will be detailed in Chapter 14).

The language/texts only hint at insights for such questions. This work seeks not to inscribe closure, but rather to retain a questioning orientation to such issues. There is, though, an acknowledgment that the spiritual discourse was a formative influence and sustaining force in the genesis of this organisation. There is also a recognition that, during the present period of routinisation, the spiritual 'will to power' contributes to a subjectivity and discursive space which is an important ingredient in the 'difference' of this organisation. The language/texts have been deconstructed to inscribe both rationalisation of spiritual impotence in the face of hegemonic power, and the constructive potentiality of fostering positive organisational relationships. The spiritual pain of the organisation's embryonic period has been compared to the spiritual contentment of its present organisation. That spirituality is a vital force impacting on the direction of this hospice organisation - a force which is valued and actively protected through the discursive practices - is affirmed and inscribed. A more detailed description of the relationship between resistance to hegemonic bureaucratic and professional discourse and the spiritual discursive practices of KHS would need further research (which will be discussed in the final chapter).

A spiritual ethical problematic

Before leaving this discussion of the impact of spirituality at the organisational level, mention needs to be made of the notion, which surfaced in the language/texts, of the possibility of ethical misuse of spiritual motivation. The following comments are situated in the understanding that all discourses are underpinned by a concealed 'will to power'. Discursive practices, such as the spiritual discourse of KHS, although privileged as positive and constructive, can be interpreted to reveal elements of control and power through an examination of the notions suppressed. As Davies clearly states,

> But any new discourse, even a discourse taught in the name of liberation from particular forms of oppression, necessarily brings with it its own set of restraints and inhibitions (1994:44).

When discussing the link between spiritual discourse and organisational practice, the assumption is not made that this link will invariably be positive. There was sufficient information arising from the language/texts to suggest that a reading of some of the notions silenced in KHS's spiritual discourse reveal elements of power which had possibilities of unhealthy practices.

This issue will now be examined in the detail offered by the participants. The expectation is *not one of conclusive findings, but of sufficient detail being available to demonstrate how these issues could be explored in further research.*

Firstly, it will be argued that the 'will to serve' of KHS's spiritual discourse can sanction altruism whilst silencing an instrumental notion of manipulation. Such spiritual discursive practices can be vulnerable to the unethical practices of seeing individuals as a means to an end.

A basic ethical concept in the discourse on ethics is the notion of respect for persons as ends in themselves. As expressed through Kantian ethical formalism, this notion suggests that ethical behaviour necessitates that we act in such a way that always treats another person as 'exalted above any price; for as such (homo noumenon) he (sic) is not to be valued as a mere means to the ends of others or even to his (sic) own ends, but as an end in himself (sic)' (Kant 1964).

Recent writers, such as Engelhardt (1991), exploring the possibility of a shared ethical discourse in a postmodern world of incommensurable value positions, where religious absolutism has been replaced by secular relativism and rationality has come under criticism, affirm this notion of respect for the individual. A foundational assumption in the ethical 'will to power', in a world of moral strangers ultimately rests on the notion of treating others as an end in themselves, not a means to an end. In the words of Engelhardt,

> Thus, even if God is silent and the project of discovering a content-full ethics fails, insofar as one is interested in engaging in ethics, that is, in resolving controversies without foundational recourse to force, one can still participate in a common moral world with moral strangers. The necessary condition for participating in that world is mutual respect, the non-use of others without their consent. This side constraint is not grounded in a value given to autonomy, liberty, or to persons, but is integral to the grammar of controversy resolution when God, facts, and reason do not provide a basis for peaceably resolving a dispute. Mutual respect is accepted because it is the one way to ground a common moral world for moral strangers without arbitrarily endorsing a particular ranking of values (1991:119).

The present reading of aspects of KHS's spiritual discourse will be premised on such notions of respect for person.

The positive aspects of spiritual motivation, both on the genesis and formation of KHS, have been acknowledged. High ideals, spiritual commitment, hard work and dedication are all ingredients which are sanctioned throughout this work as positive extensions of the spiritual 'will to power'. Some mention has been made of the emotional cost of such commitment, such as organisational 'fall out', and issues of burn out and perfectionism. Placed under erasure, however, this energising, motivating force, which is so important for the establishment and growth of this service, could also be seen to be silencing notions of manipulation. Such an understanding points to an ideological contradiction: a discourse on love and compassion which sanctions notions of holism and care contains within it the possibility of actually building organisational relationships on manipulating and using others primarily for their usefulness, (even when this is counterproductive to the individual involved). The question, as with many ethical matters, is a matter of degree, with the central question being: When does a constructive organisational policy of co-opting the skills and dedication of others, become ethically questionable practices of manipulation and a calculated use of the individual as just a means to an end?

As seen by the following language/texts, the notion of co-opting individuals of talent, professional standing and commitment, was both conscious and spiritually inscribed.

> With that inspiration we have brought in these other skilled people. We have always kept trying to bring in people with particular skills whether it is nursing or structural or financial and so with that sort of spiritual inspiration and that group of people professional committed people, and of course, the great dedication and commitment of volunteers (EQ).

> So she asked a lot of people of various backgrounds, administrative people, publicity people to actually give us advice on how we should be moving and what direction we should be moving, and how we should be publishing, how we should be conducting ourselves (EQ).

Such texts inscribe a positive and constructive motivation and outcome to such a process. Silenced is the notion of using others, of needing to repay or reward the individuals for their services. An unconditional expectation of pure giving underpins the statements.

There were just a few texts which addressed these silenced notions. As seen by the following examples, such texts suggest that, at times, the positively inscribed practice of incorporation moved to the ethically problematic area of manipulation.

> (This person) works very much on the basis of hooking people in through their personal experience. And sometimes I have problems with that because I believe there is a very fine line, a very fine line indeed between..it is very hard to express..ethical line... between asking someone to do something for you for altruistic reasons and, but really because they are doing it for you personally, because they are attracted to you personally. But the line that you cross gets into ... exploitation a hard word for it... manipulation. It is a very fine line and I felt (this person) crossed that line and that is what made me very uncomfortable with that and other people were too (EQ).

> When I started to articulate it to other people I found there was a whole group in Brisbane who had been through similar processes and who now had almost nothing to do with Karuna as a result of it because they felt they had been manipulated (EQ).

Although there were only cursory references to such a silenced dynamic in the spiritual discourse, these texts do suggest the possibility of negative practice implications of suppressed notions in spiritual *raison d'etre* of this organisation. Such a discussion provides a balance to the preceding positive exploration of the effects of KHS's spiritual discourse.

Recap and summary

To this point, this chapter has explored the ways that KHS's spiritual discourse can be seen to 'make a difference' to maintaining its ideological 'freedom' in the struggle against mainstream bureaucratic and professional notions. It has been shown that, within KHS, there is a discursive space and subjectivity, conducive to a 'gentle spirituality'. This was contrasted to the profit, income, power and status motives underpinning the discourse of biomedicine.

Such a discourse was not only seen to create and support a different 'way' of responding within the organisation, but was also shown to be effective in attracting individuals compatible with such a way of seeing and acting. The possibility of ethical misuse of such a spiritual discourse and its interrelationship with intrapsychic issues was also explored.

This examination of notions of discursive space and subjectivity within the organisation will now be explored with a specific focus on how these issues translate at the coalface of work with the client.

Spirituality at the coalface

> Language does not simply inform; it creates the very possibility for the creation of meaning environments (Mumby, 1988:102).

KHS's discourse, it is argued, creates a 'meaning environment' supportive of a democratically informed, caring organisational structure, which promotes and provides for a holistic, compassionate notion of service delivery. There is the possibility within such a discourse of holistic, compassionate, non-judgmental care at the coalface of direct work with the client. The following discussion wishes to explore that possibility by firstly, looking at the implications of such 'talk' in relation to KHS's hospice *workers* (their selection, support and how this translates into different hospice practice); secondly, examining the significance of the view of the *client* created by discursive practices of this organisation; and finally, once KHS's different worker and client space has been articulated, by *contrasting* this to the subjectivity and practice of the *biomedical* discourse in relation to patient care. The implications of such a discussion will be drawn to the experience of dying within our community.

Selecting the hospice worker

As outlined previously, KHS's spiritual discourse creates a subjectivity compatible with, and supportive of, the notion of a hospice worker in the literature.[3] KHS not only privileges and values such a subjectivity, but actively selects health professionals who demonstrate the personal characteristics which allow the expression of such inscribed ways of seeing and acting. Also, reference has been made to the discursive magnetism of KHS, which attracts, without the expenditure of its own energy, individuals of similar minds, who talk the same talk, and sanction similar values.

KHS has a clear statement of its goals and visions, seeing part of the process of respecting difference in others being the parallel responsibility of clear articulation of their own particular hospice goals and visions. This clarity contributes to the process of self-selection. The spiritual discursive practices of KHS are thus seen to be an important dynamic in the selection, attraction and valuing of the organisational members who will operate at the interface between service and clients. Such a discursive filtering mechanism, it will be argued, especially when combined with a discursive compatibility with hospice ideology, is a powerful mechanism for controlling the creation of hospice worker subjectivity.

Supporting hospice practice

The effectiveness of carrying out the work of a community based hospice depends on the hospice workers' ability to care, to communicate, to listen, to advocate, and to respect the choice of others. The work of hospice, when translated to the community setting, is one of relationship building and communication, of compassionate, non-judgmental understanding combined with a motivation to serve the holistic needs of others. The spiritual discourse of KHS, it is argued, is directly compatible with such hospice practice. As one participant expressed the connection, 'if you come from a spiritual base then you get that insight more' (EQ). There is a direct and pragmatic link between discourse and hospice practice. Participants articulated this link as 'if you do it for the right reason and the right space it flows' (EQ).

Participants suggested evidence of such a connection when they made suggestions that 'Karuna makes people feel loved' (EQ), or reported observations such as 'from what I hear about the nurses...if I was dying the Karuna nurses would be the ones I would want...unbelievably beautiful people...just full on people' (EQ).

The difference at the coalface

> You have to nurture your nurtures and care for the carers (EQ).

To travel the full circle to the beginning of this work, the support for, and valuing of, such a compassionate and sensitive subjectivity in their workers is directly related to the difference (already established) which KHS achieves in their work with clients.[4] In short, KHS attracts, supports and values qualities in their workers (be they nurse, volunteer, allied health professional or doctor) *which translates into success in achieving their expressed goals and vision of patient and family care.* In the words of one patient the members of KHS that she had contact with were,

> Compassionate loving people, very special people...wonderful care (EQ).

Of equal importance is the space such a discourse provides for the worker to use time and resources to carry out such visions and goals. There is a direct connection between talk and support for practice. This is one reason given by nurses in particular, for choosing to work at KHS rather than in mainstream organisations, as seen by the following comments,

> ...the reason I left my previous employment...wasn't supported...just didn't have the support...I do here (EQ)

It was acknowledged that 'there are individuals within all organisations who are trying to do that (i.e. support nurses to work holistically)', but the fact that this is 'the common value of all the people who are working within' KHS was considered an operative factor.[5] It is suggested that, within the spiritual discourse of KHS, workers are supported organisationally, to work holistically and compassionately with the dying.

Contextualising the difference

Participants gave examples of situations which demonstrated the difference between being at the coalface in organisations other than KHS and KHS itself. The first example was the simple act of a nurse wanting to give out her telephone number to be contacted at night. At KHS this would be seen as part of their twenty-four hour, holistic service; in other organisations this was seen as 'getting too involved', as the following statements outlines,

> (I was giving out my telephone number) because I know they were going to need it. This was seen as too involved and going to cost the organisation money. (I was told) you are getting too involved with them emotionally and shouldn't they be in hospital if they have reached that stage. Probably in four years community nursing I have been phoned six times (EQ).

> You hear professionally that there is a crisis there and professionally you are prepared to be there and that is not seen as a positive. It is seen as a burden on the community or the organisation. (With Karuna) it wouldn't be an issue (EQ).

Another example given was of the time a worker spent waiting in a doctor's surgery. At KHS this would be interpreted as important time spent as a client advocate, and in developing relationships and communication with general practitioners. In other organisations, such time was seen as wasted, as the following statement shows,

> If you spent two hours in a doctor's surgery..it would be 'What are you doing?' Where as the end result is perhaps - This is what we have achieved for our clients! But that is seen as wasting time (EQ).

Talking client subjectivity

So far, this discussion has focused on the space that the discursive practices of KHS create for the worker. Of equal importance is the 'talk' about the client. A different way of seeing the client, it is suggested, translates into a different way of relating to them.

To return in summary form to previous discussions of KHS's 'talk' about their clients, the following points emerge. Clients are not viewed individually, but in terms of their relationships to their families or significant others. The stated objective is to give full consideration to their belief systems, the meaning they are making out of their life, and their personal needs (interpreted as physio-psycho-social-spiritual needs). The individual is seen to need compassionate care and non-judgmental support in exploring their choices in coming to terms with the dying process.

The response to such a client subjectivity is compassionate, twenty four hour, holistic care which takes into account not only the patient's need for physical comfort and pain relief, but also their emotional, social and spiritual concerns. This comprehensive care extends to the family, both during the dying trajectory and as bereavement follow-up for the following year. Such holistic care necessitates that health professionals extend their focus from the purely physical to getting to know their patients 'in the fullest sense' of being human.

Central to such care is the provision of the opportunity and support for the patient to die in their own home, if that is their wish.[6] Protecting and supporting the individual's right to make choices about their lives, particularly in relation to their illness, is a fundamental value in KHS's work with the dying.[7]

The biomedical model - a very different subjectivity

> It would be disastrous to try to force holistic health care into the mould of biomedicine, whose methods are preponderantly surgical or pharmaceutical (Pelletier, 1990:38).

As outlined previously in this work (Chapter 9), this contrasts greatly with the view of the patient that is underpinned by the biomedical model.

In the biomedical model, the patient is objectified through a rational discourse based on scientific, reductionist principles, which focus on the body as 'machine'. The individual's emotional, social, and spiritual dimension are suppressed in a discourse that uses language restricted to objective 'facts' about the body.[8] Such a model 'treats diseases rather than patients' (Anaspach, 1990).[9] This is a cure oriented system, with a technological imperative predicated on doing whatever is technically possible, even if there is a low probability of benefiting the patient.[10]

The notion of person becomes depersonalised and separate from the reified body, the object of the 'clinical gaze' of biomedicine.[11] Social meanings, feelings, and even the experience of illness itself is lost in the objectifying language of biomedicine. The subjectivity of the patient in the discourse on biomedicine is that of a collection of anatomical structures and physiological processes.

The health worker's subjectivity is that of biotechnician, in a 'medical-industrial complex' that is underpinned by profit, income, status and medicocentric power. Non-technologically oriented patient care work is devalued. This often leads to an over emphasis on technology, with overused and fragmented services, where individuals must be 'cured before they die'. In our death-denying society, such a reductionist, physiological, technologically driven imperative leads to many ethical dilemmas, as witnessed by much of the research coming out of the discipline of bioethics.

When the care of the patient is situated within a medical institution, such medicocentric power and control is exacerbated by the 'top down' authority structure of the tertiary care organisation. The experience of being a patient can be one of disempowerment, fragmentation, and depersonalisation.[12]

Implications for the dying

As outlined previously, the majority in our society actually die in institutions underpinned by this scientific, biomedical discourse. Such a death is seen as lonely, institutionalised, sanitised, impersonal and controlled by technical experts. The rational scientific metaphysic of such a discourse marginalises notions of spiritual meaning making and the sacred significance of death and dying. Secular, physiological, reductionist 'talk' about 'clinical death' is the dominant discourse, which silences ideas of death as a spiritual event.

Technological developments in the medical care of the terminally ill create the possibility that the process of dying can now be a lingering, isolated and dehumanising experience in a bureaucratic medical setting, dominated by invasive technical equipment. In such a discourse, death is not a normal event, but perceived as a failure in the 'war' against disease. Invasive, aggressive, distressing interventions, rather than holistic emotional and spiritual care, characterise such a technologised, scientific response to the dying trajectory.

Control of information about the dying process usually resides with health professionals, in a disempowering social setting where the expression of autonomy and considerations of choice are difficult at best.

Different discourses: different 'ways' of responding

> The social subject that produces a statement is not an entity which exists outside of and independently of discourse, as the source of the statement,

> (its 'author'), but is on the contrary a function of the statement itself. That is, statements position subjects - those who produce them, but also those they are addressed to (Fairclough, 1992:43).

So far in this discussion, the subjectivity created by both the institutionalised biomedical discourse on dying and KHS's discourse have been compared. For both the health professional and the patient, it has been shown, these different ways of 'speaking the world' (Davies, 1994:44) translate into different ways of interacting with each other, and hence, of responding to, and experiencing death and dying.

In the light of such understanding, discourse is seen to be a powerful determinant in shaping the 'way' our society responds to issues of death and dying. The individual is constituted afresh in each discourse (Davies, 1994:4). The importance is placed on the interpretation of the individual's autonomous wishes, needs, feelings, the meaning making they bring to the dying experience, and the medical interventions considered necessary, are all context dependent: constituted by discourse.

How we die, where we die, who we die with and what medical treatment will be given are determined as much by the options made available by the different discourses as they are by any predetermined notion of individual choice.

KHS's spiritual discourse on the dying extends and enriches that notion of choice by an empowering and caring relationship between worker and patient. A sense of the caring, the willingness and the support of such a 'reality' has been expressed in the words of clients of KHS,

> They are very willing and that is the whole thing (EQ).

> I don't have a sense of imposition. Uh, I suppose, that is what the service is all about (EQ).

> Karuna gave me my choices back...I was amazed at their sincerity and compassion (Darragh, 1994).

> I am grateful to Karuna for all the support I have received especially for providing a place for me to go and people who care (Montgomery, 1995).

Such a spiritual discourse can, it is argued, can make a difference to the 'way' organisations respond to issues of death and dying.

Conclusion

It is the conclusion of this research that KHS's spiritual discourse is seen to have quite different discursive effects, in terms of whether viewed generally in organisational terms or more specifically, in relation to the impact it has at the coalface of the client.

Organisationally, the spiritual discourse (as expressed in the early dreaming of the members of the embryonic KHS) came to be dominated by the hegemonic discourse of professionalism and bureaucratisation. Interpreted as rationalisation 'both/and' a flexible response to issues of power, it was, however, acknowledged to be a potentially constructive factor in the organisational life of this service. The spiritual 'talk' was shown to provide the discursive space and subjectivity which creates, supports, and attracts ways of seeing and acting which can offer some resistance to the dehumanising aspects of biomedicine's demands. This discourse, by supporting different ways of seeing and valuing self as worker and colleague, was shown to create the spiritual space whereby individuals, in spite of the demands from more powerful discourses, can choose to act with difference.

At the interface between hospice worker and client, the spiritual discursive practices and the subjectivity such practices sanction were acknowledged as powerful mechanisms influencing hospice praxis. A direct link was drawn between spiritual discursive practices, hospice ideology and the selection, attraction, and practice of hospice workers at KHS.

The conclusion reached is that KHS's spiritual discourse can and does make a difference, particularly at the coalface of patient care. Such a discourse is constitutive: it creates and maintains a discursive space and subjectivity for both health worker and patient that inscribes an enriched notion of choice and the possibility of holistic, compassionate, non-judgmental care.

Appreciation for KHS's special 'way' can be seen in the words of their clients, who made such statements as,

> Karuna is tops just tops! (EQ).

> Well like I said, they are absolutely wonderful and they came and done everything possible to help me (EQ).

Notes

1 This is the notion of creative power within discourse articulated by Mumby (1988:63) as follows, 'power is not simply a part of organisational structure; rather, it is both medium and outcome; it is both enabling and constraining. Power, in essence, is both a product of organisational activity and the process by which activity becomes institutionally legitimated. Organisational interaction is therefore not something that takes place within the (power) structure of an organisation, but is rather the process through which structure is created, reproduced, and changed.'

2 It has already been outlined in previous discussions that members of this organisation not only expressed their 'difference' positively, but also used negative descriptive terms by stating an understanding of what they did not want to become (Chapter 4). This difference 'via negitiva' referred to a desire not to become like the biomedical model. Consequently, such a model has been used throughout this research as a basis for comparison

with KHS's spiritual discourse.

3 This relativistic notion that judgments of success (and hence selection) are relative to the background of a health system has been an ongoing assumption that underpins this work. Risjord (1993:195) reinforces this postmodern observation when he states that 'the social scientific study of medicine, therefore, does require relativism in the form of a relativism about success...Understanding a system of ideas and explaining the behavior of its adherents requires us to view the practices and ideas as the adherents do.'

4 As has already been outlined previously (Chapter 1 and Chapter 3) it was an interest created by the innumerable, enthusiastic and positive stories about KHS's difference from both clients and other health professionals which contributed to the initial motivation behind doing this research. The working assumption for this discussion is a belief that, in the face of such extensive, (and ongoing), conversational feedback on KHS's excellent, caring work with the dying, and taking into account the positive comments of present clients interviewed for this research, this community based hospice, is indeed, translating its cherished vision and values into caring, holistic, humanitarian service at the coalface of patient care. Of particular significance, in regards to this assumption, is the complete absence of any negative feedback that I have received from the many families I have spoken to who have been touched by the work of this service.

5 As stated previously, the many positive stories about KHS's work with the dying was the starting point for this work. The research curiosity initiated by these stories, focused on exploring organisational discourse, rather than on affirming the veracity of the claims of the stories of its clients. As postmodern research, this work is concerned with talk, not proof. Consequently, the focus has remained on organisational discourse and does not seek to make claims (empirical or otherwise), other than those suggested by KHS's clients about this organisation's work at the coalface of patient care. Suggestions will be made for the possibility of further research on the patient's experience, but this would be in addition to, and outside of the parameters of, the present research focus.

6 Gotay (1983:133) describes such a choice of being able to die in one's own home as encompassing 'the intangible benefits of familiar surroundings, the presence of pets and favourite possessions, the assumption by the dying person's family of primary responsibility for the provision of care, and the facilitation of family-patient companionship. It may, in short, provide what the patient wants most.'

7 This notion of choice is central to hospice philosophy and will be elaborated on in detail later in this work. As Kohut and Kohut (1984:24) state, 'It is imperative for dying patients to know and feel that they are still in command of their own lives. Maintaining their own daily schedule is a big morale booster. If a terminally ill person wants to die at home then every conceivable effort should be made to accommodate the patient and family.'

8 The biomedical model by focusing on the individuals body rather than

experience, according to Lumby (1994:2) silences 'notions of control, power, authority, helplessness, fear and change often implicit in health care situations.'

9 Lebacqz (1992:302) writes about 'the limits of medical and technical language to describe the meaning of the reality faced by the patient'. He suggests that 'illness is not merely a physical phenomenon. It is a personal phenomenon, with symbolic meaning. The symbolic meaning of illness is not totally idiosyncratic, since it will be formed in large part by cultural expectations. But it is nonetheless personal. Only the patient knows this personal side of illness.'

10 As Rinaldi and Kearl explain, 'Those trained to cure, the health-care professionals, who wanted to believe that science, when properly applied, held all of the answers, rejected dying persons as evidence of their own failure...The hospice philosophy differs radically from the dominant medical paradigm: it concentrates on care rather than cure, and encourages the terminally ill and their families to retain as much control as possible throughout the last days of life.'

11 Jecker and Self (1991:292) articulate this aspect of modern scientific medicine clearly when they write, 'The scientific paradigm that became the language and practice of medicine further reinforced a separation between physician and patient. This paradigm pictured the human being as a machine, and disease as an objective entity that interfered with the human being's mechanical functioning. Such a perspective implied that the 'ghost in the machine' was superfluous to the healing process.'

12 Understandably, as Rinaldi and Kearl explain (1990:287) 'hospice, then, can be viewed as an alternative to technological death, a reaction against the physicians' total control of the final rite-of-passage.'

13 Bioethical reflections

As outlined in the introduction, this work wishes to make a contribution to the discipline of bioethics. Consequently, the following chapter draws out the important bioethical insights and ideas that have arisen from this the preceding discussion.

To set the context for this discussion, it is important to reiterate that the bioethical issues central to this work are twofold. Firstly, there is the perplexing and ongoing question of how to respond to the increasing number of bioethical dilemmas that arise from our 'high-tech', medicalised response to issues of death and dying. Secondly, there is the epistemological concern with rationalism, and how this dominates not only our perception of end-of-life issues but also the whole nature of bioethical debate.

In response to the first issue, it will be argued that KHS's discourse contains positive and constructive notions which make an important contribution to understanding one possible ethical response to the bioethical dilemmas caused by 'high-tech' medicine in terminal illness. KHS's spiritual discourse is built around the importance of choice, based on a holistic, caring and non-judgmental respect for others. The study of such a discourse, it is suggested, provides insights into another 'way' of responding to the terminally ill that proactively deflects the very problems that bioethical reflection tries to resolve.

This idea of an alternative 'way' of responding to the dying will be extended to a consideration of the second concern (that of ethical rationalism). Central to this discussion is a concern that the rational application of principles cannot be considered outside of notions of discourse, power and subjectivity. The 'will to ethical behaviour' is not seen as a rational dynamic expressed by the application of ethical principles to difficult situations. Rather, the analysis has suggested that such an ethical 'will to power' is a function of the very discourse in which it is situated.

A postmodern approach to ethical decision-making will be proposed, and moves from the modernist notion of revering principle over context, to a concern with power, subjectivity, and discourse. Understanding difficult, end-of-life, bioethical dilemmas, it will be suggested, has as much to do with issues of discursive power and subjectivity as it does with any rational principle of ethical reasoning.

A return to the problems of high-tech end-of-life care

To contextualise the following discussion, it is important to outline in brief the end-of-life ethical problems that are of central concern to the bioethical literature.

A recurring theme of this work has been the medicalised, technologised Western response to issues of death and dying. The very emergence of bioethics as a discipline, it has been explained, was a direct response to the difficult ethical issues such a 'way' of caring for the terminally ill created (Miller and Rahr, 1983:268). What, then, are the problems of high-tech care?

Dominating the bioethical literature is a concern with how to respond ethically, when humans are 'linked up' to technology which is only prolonging life artificially, with a very poor or negative quality of life. In the words of Lockwood (1985:2), such a 'hi-tech angst' centres on the reality that 'modern 'hi-tech' medicine is now capable of keeping patients alive in circumstances in which they would previously have died and in which it would generally have been considered a blessing that they should die'. Such technology leads to a 'pandora's box' of ethical questions, including the exploration of requests to disconnect ventilators and life support systems of the terminally ill (Brock, 1989; Edwards and Tolle, 1993; Fullbrook, 1992; Fisher and Raper, 1990); a concern with notions of treatment futility (Jecker, 1991:7; Truog, Brett and Frader, 1993); efforts to define the whole notion of death (Brock, 1989; Campbell et al., 1992:109; Downie and Calman, 1987:207; Singer, 1994; Veatch, 1976:46); if and when nutrition and hydration can ethically be removed from those in permanent vegetative state (Boisaubin, 1993; Finnis, 1993); the right to refuse treatment (Auer, 1990:69; Chervenak and McCullough, 1991; Scarlett, 1994; Tonti-Filippini, 1992; Otlowski, 1995; Wear and Brahams, 1991; Wreen, 1991; Otlowski, 1995) and a concern about the effect of such technology on the human experience of dying (Cassell, 1991; Kass, 1991; Raffin, Shurkin and Sinkler, 1989).

In a medical milieu where it is easier to start life support systems than withdraw them (Bedel and Delbanco, 1986; Cassell, 1991), considerable bioethical reflection centres on the use and abuse of 'Not for Resuscitation Orders'(also referred to as Do Not Resuscitate (DNR) or No Code) (Bedell and Delbanco, 1986; Blackhall, 1987; Evans and Brody, 1985; Haines, Zalcberg and Buchanan, 1990; Johnstone, 1994 :397; Scofield, 1991a; Tomlinson and Brody, 1988; Torda and Berber, 1989). The concern is to avoid the experience of a distressing invasive futile treatment for those in the dying trajectory. With an increasing awareness that heroic measures such as cardiopulmonary resuscitation (CPR) were only useful for those without underlying fatal diseases (patients with chronic conditions rarely survived)

(Haines et al., 1990:226). Bioethical guidelines were developed, which emphasised a reflective consideration in the use of such technologies and a respect for the autonomous wishes of the patient receiving the intervention (Blackhall, 1987; Stanley and Reid, 1989). Slowly, such ethical reflection has been enshrined in the legal right to refuse such unwanted heroic measures (Otlowski, 1995:36).

Ethical and legal safeguards to such invasive technology have been sought through notions of advanced directives or living wills (Annas, 1991; Bok, 1976; Downie and Calman, 1987:209; Emanuel, 1991; Gillon, 1988; Greaves, 1989; Stuparich, 1992:10; Veatch, 1976:182) and legislative reform (Otlowski, 1995).

Bioethical concern about such invasive scientific medical interventions does not end at death but extends, because of a medical technology known as organ transplantation, to the use of body parts after death. With regards to this 'hi-tech' process, ethical debate focuses on such issues as the harvesting and ownership of body parts (Andrews, 1986; Johnstone, 1994:421; Mandel, 1993; Teo, 1991), defining death (Bayertz, 1992; Pearson, 1993b), safeguarding informed consent for recipients and donors (Singer et al., 1989), and the emotional experience of organ transplantation for those involved (Sherson, 1991).

At a time when there is a realisation of the limits to the health care dollar (Charlesworth, 1993:108), the enormous costs of end-of-life technology leads to important ethical questions about cost containment and resource allocation (Aaron and Schwartz, 1985; Brody, 1987; Boyle, 1984; Goodman, 1991; Joseph, 1993; Mehlman, 1986; Menzel, 1990; Morreim, 1987; Williams, 1974; Raffin, Shurkin and Sinkler, 1989; Veatch, 1988). The high costs of medical technology in terminal care is especially worrying in view of the inverse relationship of cost to survival in intensive care units (Bayer et al, 1983;), the excessive ordering of unnecessary tests (Bates and Linder Pelz, 1987; Wong et al., 1983), and a concern that very expensive technology is indeed replacing a reliance on personal human caring (Relman, 1980; Saunders and Baines, 1983; Veatch, 1976).

The overriding concern in such bioethical reflection has been on the dehumanising experience of dying in the medicalised, sanitised, alienated world of the tertiary care institutional setting. The ethical safeguards to resolving such 'hi-tech' angst have centred on advancing notions of patient autonomy, informed consent, and confidentiality (Campbell, Gillett and Jones, 1992; Gillett, 1989; Lockwood, 1985) in a rational discourse which operates on principles of autonomy, beneficence, non-maleficence and justice (Johnstone, 1994; Mappes and Zembaty, 1991; Mitchell and Lovat, 1991).

In summary, it can be seen that bioethical dilemmas arise from a highly technologised, medical approach to dying in an institutional milieu which fosters intervention with insufficient consideration of the human cost. The issues on the bioethical agenda are directly related to the modernist, biomedical, scientific discourse on death and dying. The 'talk' of bioethics is in many ways, an extension of the reductionist physiological 'talk' of biomedicine, incorporating concepts of ventilators, life support systems, treatment futility, rights to refuse or withdraw from treatment, the legitimacy of organ transplantation, the harvesting and ownership of body parts, not for resuscitation orders, and cardiopulmonary resuscitation. Such language focuses on, and is restricted to, institutions dominated by the hegemonic power of the medical profession.

The solutions to such dilemmas are explored from within the very discourse (biomedicine) which created the problems in the first place. Ethical reflection translates into the development of guidelines (e.g. guidelines to cardiopulmonary resuscitation) and the framing of documents (e.g. consent forms) which presupposes that biomedicine is *the* way to respond to terminal illness and death.

With the central guiding principle of autonomy (Callahan, 1994:28; Charlesworth, 1993; Downie and Calman, 1987:51), protection for patient rights is developed at the micro-level at the interface between patient and health professional. The patient is still situated within the awesome power of the biomedical discourse. To understand an alternative approach to bioethical issues, the discursive power of biomedicine needs to be described.

The power of the biomedical discourse

> 'You see, you start from a completely false position. No sooner does a patient come to you than you begin to do all his thinking for him. After that, the thinking's done by your standing orders, your five-minute conferences, your programme, your plan and the honour of your medical department. And once again I become a grain of sand, just like I was in the camp. Once again nothing depends on me'.
>
> 'The clinic obtains written consent from every patient before every operation,' Donstsova reminded him (Solzhenitsyn, 1971:86).

A great deal of sociological literature has been written on the power and dominance of biomedicine, highlighting the asymmetry between physician and patient. From the early 1950s, structuralist sociological descriptions articulated the role of medicine as an agent of social control (Parsons, 1951). By defining who could be ascribed to the 'sick role' (and hence exempt from societal expectations of responsibility), doctors were seen as both powerful over others and instrumental in maintaining the power of the social system. Such hegemonic power was later theorised as an extension of the physicians' professional authority: that is, authority based on professional autonomy or the freedom from outside control (Freidson 1970). According to Freidson, such authority both defines 'what illness really is' and exercises the right 'to create illness as an official social role' (Freidson, 1970:205-6). In short, the medical profession was seen to be in a powerful role in both defining and creating the experience of ill health.

Writers such as Zola (1974) conceptualised such power and dominance as an insidious process known as 'medicalisation', through which biomedicine's 'technical, scientific, objective' assumptions assert their relevance to every sphere of human activity. Such a medicalised approach to life experiences allows problems to be discussed only in medical terms, with only medical solutions permitted (Bransen, 1992:98). Under the rubric of caring, such medicalisation is understood by many authors to expand the dominance and social control role of biomedicine (Illich, 1976; Ehrenreich and Ehrenreich, 1978; Waitzkin, 1989; Waitzkin and Stoeckle, 1976). Illich's work (1976) extended this notion of medicalisation of life to include the medicalisation of death. His foreboding research predicts a 'medical nemesis' where the very power attributed to modern medicine is seen to be the creator of clinical, social and cultural iatrogenesis (1976:127). Illich states,

> Professionally organised medicine has come to function as a domineering moral enterprise that advertises industrial expansion as a war against all suffering. It has thereby undermined the ability of individuals to face their reality, to express their own values, and to accept inevitable and often irremediable pain and impairment, decline and death (1976:127-8).

Critical theorists such as Waitzkin (1989) acknowledge the importance of understanding this power of biomedicine and, along with other Marxists analysts (Navarro, 1976), conceptualise an instrumental connection between this power and maintaining the status quo of capitalist society. Waitzkin states,

> In accepting the present context as given, and in remaining silent about collective political action, medical discourse encourages consent by rendering social change unthinkable. This latter accomplishment of medicine may be its main contribution to social control (1989:236).

Translating such notions to discourse, writers such as Mishler challenge the biomedical model as but one representation or picture of reality (1981:1). With research based on transcripts of medical encounters, the doctor is shown to typically dominate physician/patient communication by steering conversation to technical concerns. Speaking of a dichotomy between the 'voice of medicine' (articulated by the doctor) and the 'voice of the life world' (spoken by the patient), Mishler (1984) argues that the technical, bioscientific, medical voice dominates over the social and emotional concerns of the patient.

Within postmodern writing, perhaps the most significant influence on the notion of the dominance of the biomedical discourse has been Foucault's work on the relationship between knowledge, power and social control. Foucault marks the development of biomedical dominance 'precisely from the moment clinical experience became the anatomo-clinical gaze' (1973:145). This idea of the 'clinical gaze' refers to the reductionist, scientific way the medical profession came to view all disease and ill health: the individual is viewed only in physiological terms. According to Foucault (1973), in Western industrial society, such a scientific medical perspective, associated as it is with the prestige of the medical profession institutionalised through the 'birth of the clinic', became a hegemonic discourse which marginalised, or even excluded, other forms of knowledge. Through his writings which link such knowledge with power, Foucault (1980) argues that claims to objective, scientific, medical knowledge are disguised as claims to truth, by experts claiming ownership of such a dominant discourse. This Foucaultian notion of the 'discourses of truth' affirms the old aphorism that 'knowledge is power'. Using the metaphor of a panopticon, Foucault (1973) posits that the power of the modernist medical 'gaze' translates into surveillance, scrutiny and control.

In view of this brief overview of our theoretical understanding of the power of the biomedical discourse, it is strongly argued that no reflection on the bioethical issues arising from within such a discourse can be considered independently of such issues of power. But what do these ideas of the power of the biomedical discourse mean for the patient who is dying in hospital?

Translating the power asymmetry to the institutional setting

Within the hospital, the identity of the patient is so dominated by institutionalised medical power that all behaviour and access to other people is directed by the demands of medical treatment (Hart, 1985, 1985:105). By using Goffman's (1968) ideas of a total institution, hospitals can be understood as places where the patient is stripped of social identity, and reinscribed (through such acts as form filling, dressing in hospital garb, removal of personal possessions, lack of contact with significant others and the imposition of hospital rules and rituals) with the passive role of being just a body ready for bio-medical processing. Through the rules, regulations, and standard operating procedures, hospitals demand a passivity and submissiveness of patients (Gerteis, 1993:33). As Hart explains,

> In a hospital setting doctors possess much more power to make patients conform to their ideal requirements of unquestioning, passive obedience. The rituals of admission seemed designed to communicate this change in the balance of power in the sick role (Hart, 1985:106).

In the hospital, a patient's life is totally disrupted by the routines of an organisation which are designed for efficiency and the needs of others, with only a limited interest in the individual as physiological identity (Roth, 1979:421). Most people are consequently very glad to leave the hospital setting (ibid).

According to the research of Gerteis (1993), the most common sensation of those undergoing hospital treatment was a loss of sense of autonomy and control. In the words of one of the patients interviewed,

> In the role of the patient, you are once again stripped of your control, regardless of how good the hospital is, and I think that's the biggest issues that I've had with being sick (1993:33).

Interesting, and important for the bioethical implications of this study, is the notion that these expectations of institutional control and patient passivity are so routine a part of hospital life that this dynamic is rarely questioned. In the words of one patient who was asked to comment on the adjustment to hospitalisation,

> 'Nothing really', he replied, 'except do as I'm told. There's no force, they haven't forced you into any adjustment whatsoever except that you obey the rules. If they want more blood they take more blood' (Gerteis, 1993:33).

Taussig (1980), who describes the sick person as a 'dependent and anxious person, malleable in the hands of the doctor and the health system', views this routine acceptance of control as a reification of the actual process of manipulation 'concealed by the aura of benevolence' (1980:4). Such a dynamic can also be understood through notions of discourse by using Fairclough's ideas on naturalisation (1989:91; 1985:753). In these terms, such an acceptance of control would be viewed as the power of the medical discourse dominating the hospital organisation to such an extent that it has become natural and legitimate: simply *the* way of organising the healing experience. Such discourse would be seen as naturalised, no longer one of several ways of acting, but rather just common sense.

In summary, it has been shown that the hospital experience for the patient is one of a loss of social identity in a world of control and domination by health professionals whose primary interest in the person is the treatment of their physical symptoms. May shares a similar conclusion when he writes,

> Despite its indisputable technological advantages over the home, the hospital exacts a high price both psychologically and financially. Psychologically, it gnaws - with its alien machines, rhythms, language, and routines - at that identity which a person previously maintained in the outside world. The patient must surrender his customary *control* of his world not only to the disease but to those who fight against it. His capacity for *savouring* his world is also numbed by the disease and by those procedures imposed upon him in the fight against it - diet, drugs, X-rays, surgery, nausea-inducing therapy, and sleeping potions. Finally, his capacity for *communication* with his world erodes as he loses his social role. Just as disease rips him out of his usual place in the community and makes him feel less secure in his dealings with fellows, the procedures of the hospital remind him acutely of this loss by placing him in the hands of professionals - the nurse and the doctor- precisely those who seem unassailably secure in their own identities (1991:145).

It is in such a milieu that bioethical dilemmas arise and the predominant response of bioethics is to suggest reflective but rational solutions at the micro-level of the interface between doctor and patient. As will be seen through the following discussion, this rational approach is called Principlism.

Rationalism and the 'Georgetown mantra'

> Rational argument can only ever get us from our starting point to our conclusion: and if our starting point is mistaken, so may our conclusions be, however impeccable our logic (Lockwood, 1985:7).

The discipline of bioethics has been historically based on the normative enterprise of Principlism (Fox, 1994). Principlism is a rational, deductive, philosophical enterprise, exemplified by such texts as the *Principle of Biomedical Ethics,* by Beauchamp and Childress (1983), which gives central place in ethical deliberation and justification to a quartet of principles - respect for autonomy,[1] beneficence,[2] non-maleficence,[3] and justice[4] (the so called 'Georgetown Mantra')[5] (Callahan, 1988; Engelhardt and Wildes, 1994:135; Kieffer, 1979:45; Lustig, 1992:487; Mappes and Zembaty, 1991; Veatch, 1989).

This rule-based enterprise of Principlism is described by Veatch (1989:6), one of the leading authors in medical ethics as,

> the enterprise of disciplined reflection on moral intuitions and moral choices. It often begins with intuitions and long-held convictions. It attempts to compare them for consistency, to formulate rules of conduct accounting for our considered judgments and to articulate general principles that might underlie these judgments and rules.

Although Principlism still holds a central place in the discourse of bioethics, there has been, in recent years, some challenge to this position (Alderson, 1991; DeGrazia, 1992; Nicholoson, 1994; Williams, 1985). This theory based, rationalistic approach has been criticised for being ossified and formulaic and hence irrelevant to the 'complexity and joyful variety of real life' (Nicholson, 1994:269).[6] Williams (1985:197) critiques this method as 'governed by a dream of a community of reason that is too far removed.' Indeed, the very model of Principlism, itself has been forwarded as the cause of the 'sluggishness', or lack of advancement of bioethical theory (DeGrazia, 1992:512). Authors such as Alderson (1991) attack the emphasis on abstractions and rules because of its illusion of neutrality which ignores issues of human emotions and power (Alderson, 1991). Such criticism shares the concern of this analysis that this rationalistic approach to bioethics does little to 'tackle the issues of where power lies, and how it is used, in health care' (Nicholoson, 1994 :272).

As articulated previously, a central concern for bioethical epistemology in the context of postmodernity is the insuperable difficulties of applying ethical principles in the vacuum of a universal moral narrative (Engelhardt and Wildes, 1994; Wildes, 1992;485).[7] The application of such principles evoke difficult and, as yet, unresolved (or perhaps unresolvable) problems in relation to the unlimited possibility of incommensurable ethical positions in a democratic, pluralistic, multicultural society. This problem of relativism is acknowledged as a moral conundrum worth exploring, rather than as a justification to retreat to an absolutist position based on the foundational assumptions of Principlism. Principlism presupposes rationality and a deductive logic. A postmodern interpretation of reality shuns such logic for an understanding that is polycentric, often paradoxical, and sometimes *aporetic.*[8] The modernist promise of an unambiguous rational answer to ethical problems which can be deduced from a set of regularly repeated moral principles is challenged as a simplified substantive rationality.[9] Such a rationality avoids facing the complexity of the construction of reality through power of/in discourse, subjectivity, and the multiplicity of metaphysical perspectives. In such a view, the substantial rationality of principlism may be charged as being just the discourse of predominantly male, middle class, Western academics.[10] Indeed, Fox (1994) characterises such a rationality as intellectually provincial, morally chauvinistic, and culturally myopic.[11] This disbelief in the modernist project of clarification of ethical problems through the application of principles is clearly expressed by Bauman (1993:10) when he writes,

> The foolproof - universal and unshakeably founded - ethical code will never be found; having singed our fingers once too often, we know now what we did not know then, when we embarked on this journey of exploration: that a non-aporetic, non-ambivalent morality, an ethics that is universal and 'objectively founded', is a practical impossibility; perhaps also an oxymoron, a contradiction in terms.

This work not only accepts this critique of Principlism, but wishes to take up the challenge of exploring alternative 'ways' of arriving at ethical insights. In place of the substantial rationality of Principlism situated in the modernist confidence in reason, this bioethical research offers a contribution (as will be detailed in the following discussion) based on notions of discourse, power, and subjectivity. In view of the complexity of issues under discussion, however, it is important for clarity of argument, to pause momentarily in the development of these ideas to draw together the many lines of thought explored so far.

Drawing the threads together

> Slowly we are learning that the wielding of our high-tech guns is not to be equated with doing everything possible. This involves a different approach, a treating of the whole person, a negotiation and consultation and a tailoring of treatment to the individual. It involves making ourselves available to answer people's questions, sitting by the bedside, drawing diagrams, talking to angry relatives and above all admitting that we have not power to cure - that we are not God (Cassidy, 1991:17).

To this point, the central concerns of end-of-life bioethical issues have been articulated and situated within the dominant discourse of highly technologised medicocentric institutional power. There can be no understanding of such bioethical issues, it is argued, unless cardinal importance is given to the implications of this dynamic of power.

Bioethical issues have been shown to be directly linked to, and, indeed, evolved out of, our institutionalised, medicalised approach to death. The present response to such problems operates within the biomedical discourse and is consequently is an extension of the 'talk' and practices of such a discourse. Patient autonomy is discussed, consent forms are developed, resuscitation guidelines are written, living wills and the power of attorney are legally sanctioned, and hospital ethic committees explore difficult cases. Meanwhile, the patients continue to enter the disempowering, alienating world of high tech medicine, driven by the professional domination of medicine and the financial stakes of the medical industrial complex.

Within such a medicocentric and technologised milieu, the complex bioethical issues that arise are addressed by the application of a set of rationalistic principles to dilemmas after they arise.

Such a view of bioethical discourse can be seen as 'band-aid' tactics, offering some protection to the patient but little resistance to the hegemonic system. Such a bioethical discourse may, indeed, further legitimate the system by incorporating a publicly acknowledged ethical response. In a discourse where power is reified and disguised under the rubric of caring, the work of bioethicists may actually contribute to the naturalisation of such power (as the previous quote by Solzhenitsyn (1971:86) intimated).[12]

The contribution of this analysis is to suggest that there is another response to such end-of-life bioethical issues. This response is to step outside the biomedical system and the modernist rational approach to ethics. By so doing, it is possible to look at different 'ways' of responding to the problems associated with caring for the dying. KHS's spiritual discourse provides one such example of a different 'way' of looking after the terminally ill. It is proposed that a postmodern examination of this discourse could significantly inform the present bioethical challenge to Principlism.

A caveat to this particular bioethical interpretation is that it arises from postmodern research and hence, there is no expectation that the ideas generated can be enlarged to a bioethical theory about dying that can be simply applied to any, many or all situations involving the terminally ill. This research is local, ad hoc and contextual: it is based on the work of one community based hospice service (KHS) at one point in time. There are many psycho-social and spiritual factors which combined to make this service different. These factors (which have been detailed throughout this research) may or may not be able to be duplicated. It is my hope, however, that the insights gained (both epistemological and ethical) may be able to be applied to other situations involving bioethical dilemmas (on the full continuum from birth to death). Equally, it is hoped that the voice of experience of those engaged in forming this service may eventually contribute to the development of such services elsewhere.

What then is the perception of KHS's different 'way'? And what are the conclusions reached about the contribution of this discourse to bioethics?

Finding another 'way': the contribution of KHS

This discussion of the contribution of the discourse of KHS to bioethical reflection does not seek to repeat in detail the many ideas that have arisen out of this research. The discussion will be built upon the preceding exploration of notions of discourse, power, and subjectivity in relation to the discourse of KHS, and will focus on the importance of KHS's commitment to providing choices for the terminally ill.

The appropriateness of this decision to focus specifically on the whole notion of choice is strongly held for the following four reasons. Firstly, the central guiding principle in bioethics is the value and importance of individual autonomy (Charlesworth, 1993; Johnstone, 1994:91; Mitchell and Lovat, 1991:25; Pellegrino and Thomasma, 1988:3). This analysis is situated in the discipline of bioethics, and the central concern of that enterprise is a disciplined reflection on the nature of choice, in particular, moral choice. As Veatch[13] explains,

> Ethics is the enterprise of disciplined reflection on the moral intuitions and moral choices that people make...In fact it is the very nature of medical decisions that value choices must be made constantly. To decide to pursue a particular course is to decide that it is better or more right than available alternatives, and deciding that something is better or more right means making value judgments. Many of those value judgments involve ethical choices. Thus for people to make choices about their health is at its core an exercise in ethics (1989:2-3).

As will be witnessed by the following discussion, the ethical concern with choice is underpinned in bioethics by the value of autonomy. In short, the notion of autonomous choice and the discipline of bioethics are intricately and centrally linked. Consequently, an exploration of KHS's creation of choice situates this work at the very heart of bioethics where it is meant to be.

Secondly, respect for individual choice is a central ethical tenet of another major discipline central to this work, that of hospice/palliative care (Jeffrey, 1993:5). The exploration of autonomous choice consequently situates this work in the discipline of hospice/palliative care, which is a primary aim of undertaking this research.

Thirdly, the notion of choice was raised regularly and stated clearly by participants to be at the heart of what they perceived as important in their work. This is affirmed by KHS's 'Values and Vision Statement', which states that,

> We are actively involved in the promotion and support of choice and control by terminally ill people and their loved ones. We affirm our clients' ability to choose what is right and best for them.

The voices of those involved in KHS clearly state that the provision of choice is not only an issue, but a most important issue. This research respects that statement.

Fourthly, the whole notion of choice surfaced through the interpretation of this analysis as a central theme to the author. Such a theme resonates with the profound interest in exploring alternatives in working with the dying which is a motivating factor underpinning the energy for this work. To the author, the provision (for those who wish it) of the opportunity to die in the comfort and familiarity of one's own home rather than in the impersonal and frightening technological environment of a hospital ward is a concern so profound it moves beyond intellectual curiosity. The exploration and privileging as important of such a choice becomes, for the author, a moral imperative, not an intellectual decision.

A postmodern approach to research incorporates an understanding of my 'will to power' and a consequent respect for including a self-reflexive understanding of the interpretation and analysis of data. In view of such an understanding, it is acknowledged that this focus on choice is not inevitable, but rather situates the author in the philosophical tradition of a liberal, democratic society which has its historical roots in the liberalism of such writers as Locke, Rousseau, Bentham, Mill, and Kant (Russell, 1946). Equally such a focus highlights my location at the cross roads of the disciplines of bioethics and hospice/palliative care, which, as has been explained, have their origins in a philosophical concern and commitment to exploring the notion of autonomous choice. However, as this work is concerned with notions of discourse, the liberal assumption is not made that the idea of autonomy can be reified to the abstract level of a principle which can, somehow independent of the every day 'talk' of an organisation, be arbitrarily and rationally imposed on any situation. Rather autonomy is seen (as will be discussed later in this chapter) as a function of the very discourse in which it is notionally embedded. In short, the notion of autonomous choice is historically acknowledged, respected, and suspected at the same time.

In summary, this work brings both an acknowledgement that the whole notion of autonomous choice is historically and intellectually situated, and a suspicion that such a notion is restricted and confined to how it is used within discourse. As will be explored in a later discussion, the 'both/and' orientation of the postmodern approach will be used to argue that the idea of autonomy can be deeply respected by the author as a constructive and empowering notion which has important implications for our work with the dying 'both/and' seen as a dangerous notion that is, to a large degree, dependent on how it is used in discourse.

'Karuna is choice'

> In their own homes...they are the boss...they are in control...not close to a lot of technology and not caught up in that hype...there is nothing like being in your own surroundings, being in your own bed (EQ).

The word autonomy is derived from the Greek *autos* (meaning self) and *nomos* (meaning rule) (Johnstone, 1994:91), and so implies the notion of self-rule, or the individual's right to determine their own actions. Underpinning such a principle is a democratic respect for the life space of each individual, their uniqueness and fundamental importance: in short, autonomy is based on a broader principle of respect for persons.

The concept of autonomy is closely associated with the democratic notion of freedom, as can be seen in the definition by Shenkin (1991:78): stated as 'the capacity to think, decide and act on the basis of such thought and decision freely and independently and without ..let or hindrance'. The point is that the ideal of autonomy incorporates a respect for the seemingly 'wrong' decisions of others. As Beauchamp and Walters (1982:27) state,

> Insofar as an autonomous agent's actions do not infringe on the autonomous actions of others, that person should be free to perform whatever action he or she wishes (presumably even if it involves considerable risk to himself and even if others consider the action to be foolish).

Bioethical discourse gives primacy to this principle of autonomy. In the medical setting, the protection of the patient's autonomy is enshrined in such rational processes as information giving, obtaining informed consent, engaging in patient advocacy, and articulating patient rights (Johnstone, 1994). This is a rational framework based on the assumption that if the correct information is given then the right decision will be reached.

As important as these rational processes are, they are limited by two important sociological factors: firstly, the enormous power of the medical milieu to impose control over even the most assertive patient; and secondly, the fact that autonomous choice will always be limited to the actual choices available. A terminally ill patient situated within the power of the discursive context of the institutional medical setting may, for example, accept the offer of 'heroic' treatment measures. However, even when the full details of the treatment are given, if the patient is unaware of the alternative of being supported at home, is seeking the doctor's approval, or is afraid of refusing treatment because of a fear of medical abandonment (Jecker and Schneiderman, 1995:153), then the decision to accept treatment may have as much to do with the negative factors associated with refusing treatment as with the positive factors of accepting. Is such decision making compliance or autonomous choice? In a medical system where the individual 'is cured before they are allowed to die', such 'choices' are a regular occurrence. Such factors as patient intimidation in a hospital setting (Field and James, 1993), the overwhelming complexity of the modern medical system (Seffrin et al., 1991:1785), the vulnerability created through the high and hopeful expectations individuals bring to the medical encounter (Dutton, 1988; McGrath, 1993; McGrath, 1995), the feelings of helplessness and loss of control a patient experiences in the hospital setting (Gerteis, 1993:33), a fear of abandonment (McGrath, 1995), and the dependent and anxious state of the sick individual (Taussig, 1980:4) can be interpreted as powerful pressures on the patient which cause them to accept the treatment offered.

The discourse of bioethics places a great deal of emphasis on the importance of truth telling and information giving in ensuring informed consent to medical treatments offered. Although it is acknowledged that these are important, indeed imperative processes, it is also suggested that such a response to protecting patient autonomy is still very rationalistic, which assumes that information can be held as truth and that rationality can lead to good decisions. Such an approach does not sufficiently take into account the emotional and power issues involved.

In comparison to this,[14] in the discourse of KHS, the bioethical concept of autonomy is translated into a *more pragmatic notion of providing 'choice', which incorporates an understanding of the role of power and the emotions.* It will be argued that such an interpretation of autonomy by the *active creation of choices has much to contribute to our understanding of bioethical issues.*

KHS's philosophy was succinctly expressed by one participant as, 'basically what I see Karuna as being is offering people a choice' (EQ). The provision of such choice includes the standard bioethical safeguards of information giving as seen by the statement that KHS nurses 'offer them (patients and their families) the best options, best information, and what the likely outcome of those options is. Then, they can make whatever choices' (EQ).

But more importantly, the *discourse of KHS is actively and imaginatively concerned with creating a situation in which a patient and their family are provided with as many alternatives as possible.* The emphasis is on providing, not only information, but also education, and physical, emotional, social and spiritual support. The discourse of KHS is concerned with the provision of 'choice by doing' not just by talking or information giving. Such 'choice by doing' translates into twenty-four hour holistic care with the involvement of volunteers for practical and psycho-social support, community based nursing and medical care, and counselling. The dying person is seen in the context of their family or significant others. Their needs are interpreted as not just physical but psycho-social and spiritual. Most importantly, such a response is based on a non-judgmental respect for the individual's desire to handle problems in their own way, even when such choices may not seem the right way to others. Such choice incorporates the possibility that the patient can die in their own home.

Most significantly for this discussion, such respect for choice is not just confined to the limited offerings of the treatment plan of a single medical institution, but rather, is based on empowering the patient to explore options most suited to themselves. This was expressed in the words of one participant as 'the people involved need to be open to walking that individual's journey and not coming in with any of their own judgements' (EQ). Whilst KHS can offer the remarkable option for the individual to die in their own home, there is no expectation that this will always be viewed as desirable by the patient and their family, as seen by the following statement,

> We don't push any point, we try not to push people to stay at home, we try not to push a message to people...that there is one right way of doing things (EQ).

The staff of KHS do support people in their own homes, but equally they also make referrals to institutional care, if the patient so desires. The point is that, in the discourse of KHS, the notion of patient autonomy is not concerned with just information giving and the filling out of consent forms, but is rather a whole orientation to 'empowerment' that is inclusive and respectful of the many paths the individual may wish to follow. Such a process of empowerment is not only demonstrated by the practical assistance to die in their own home, but by a respectful support to move to institutional care if that is the choice. In the discourse of KHS the effect of control moves from the health professional to the patient, as can be seen by the following comment,

> (At) Karuna the client is in control. The nursing staff or the medical staff is not in control...(that is) why they chose Karuna (EQ).

Interestingly, studies of medical power (Cassell, 1991a) indicate that the power asymmetry is reversed when the patient is in their own home. The health professional defers to the power of the client when the interaction is conducted in the domestic sphere rather than the institutional setting. As Hart (1985:107) explains,

> As long as a person is at home, even if bedridden, there is some control over daily routine. In the hospital all vestiges of personal power are removed as the person becomes subject to the unpredictable whims of staff.

For the *work of KHS, the notion of autonomy is not a bioethical principle to be applied to difficult situations, but an everyday 'way' of responding to the needs of the client and their family.* This 'everyday response' (as has been outlined in detail in Chapter 12) is situated in, and supported by, KHS's spiritual discourse.

Such a spiritual discourse was shown to be actively creating and supporting both the discursive space for holistic care of the dying and a subjectivity for a compassionate and tolerant hospice worker. Not only was the KHS way of 'speaking the world' seen to attract and support individuals who sanction a loving, caring and gentle way of relating to each other and the families they work with, it also informed a client subjectivity based on a psycho-social-spiritual interpretation of their needs.

In such a discourse, choice is interpreted in a full appreciation of the individual's needs and the meaning they bring to, and are making out of, their dying experience. Choice is not predicated on the notion of the narrow options of what can and can not be physiologically or medically done to the body. Most importantly, KHS's spiritual discourse not only provides the discursive space for a holistic interpretation of choice, it also creates and supports a compassionate, non-judgmental, worker subjectivity necessary for translating and protecting such client choice.

KHS's discourse on choice, not only embraces their orientation to client care, but also includes an acceptance that such a 'way' of operating may not be suitable for everyone. As articulate as they are in expressing their ideas of choice, members of this service accept that even their discourse of choice may not be suitable to the many who seek the 'hi-tech fix'. In the words of one participant, 'Karuna is not for everyone' (EQ). Although, as the following text shows, they do sometimes support individuals who wish to straddle both worlds,

> ...it doesn't mean to say that the people that we look after aren't still searching for that high tech...that is part of it, I think they are, a lot of our younger families are, people in their 30s, 40s, 50s, children..still looking for the promise of high tech (EQ).

KHS, as has been already outlined, operates on a discursive magnet that attracts those comfortable with the discourse. This is not a proselytising organisation but one comfortable with the Taoist notion of going with the flow. The word choice in such a discourse infers a deep acceptance that becoming involved in the very discourse itself is a matter of choice. The same cannot be said for the biomedical discourse with its power and control reified and depoliticised to a discourse of the normal.

But isn't choice a dated notion of Liberalism?

This interpretation of the discourse of KHS as providing choice could be seen as a simplistic modernist view based on outdated liberal notions. Certainly, the ideology of autonomous choice central to bioethics can be historically situated as originating from the liberal political theory of John Stuart Mill. His essay, *On Liberty,* stands as a central reference for autonomy in the literature on bioethics (Charlesworth, 1993:15).[15]

The postmodern approach to discourse and power would suggest that the 'will to power' underpinning any discourse, even that of KHS, is in an active relationship to defining what can and cannot be said, and what can and cannot be done. Such power operates to restrict and define choice. In such a view, the suspicion would be that the discourse of KHS, rather than extending choice, would only be engaged in imposing its own set of discursive rules and expectations. The notion of choice, so interpreted, could be viewed as an illusion; a reification of KHS's desire to control but with a different (albeit constructive) agenda.

The interpretative position chosen is situated in the 'both\and' postmodern perspective. It is acknowledged that there can be parallel possibilities of both a constraining 'will to power' and the extension of choice. The following discussion will focus on the extension and provision of choice, whilst the restricting impact of KHS's 'will to power' is suggested as a useful focus for further research.

As has been detailed in earlier chapters, the majority of people in our society die in institutional care. The trajectory towards death, it has been shown, is a time of greatly increased medical and nursing care. The realistic provision of the option to die at home necessitates considerable resources to meet the range of physio-psycho-social-spiritual needs of the dying individual and their carer(s). Without the services of KHS (or organisations similar to them) there cannot be a choice to die at home. Pain relief, symptom control, and the management of death will stay within the institutional setting. For those who value the opportunity to die at home (and the assumption is not made that everyone will), the very existence of such a service *will provide such a choice*. So viewed, the choice KHS offers is not an intellectual illusion but a realistic, practical option.

As has already been outlined, this choice includes not only the opportunity to die at home, but extends to a respect for each individual to chose their own path in dying. Hence, KHS will equally support the patient to die in an institutional setting if that is their wish, with the flexibility of continuing care if the patient changes their mind and wishes to return home again. The important point is, that it is the actual discourse of KHS which is engaged in socially constructing such choices and pathways. It is acknowledged that such choices are still made within the space of already existing discourses, and hence will be restricted and defined to a large degree by these discourses. However, it is the strong conclusion that the discourse of KHS is still, to a large degree, in the act of creating the discursive space for extending choice. As this is postmodern research with an interest in local, ad hoc solutions, rather than a teleological notion of social reform or a grand theory of progress, this humble demonstration of the ability to extend choice is deemed important and valued.

This does not negate the inevitability that, even within this discourse of choice, power and control are exercised, with ideas privileged and notions silenced. Even in caring relationships messages are exchanged about legitimate ways of acting and appropriate responses to demands. The language/texts only suggest interesting possibilities worth exploring, rather than any firm conclusions. As suggested in the next chapter, exploring these possibilities would need the focus of further research.

A central question for such further research would be an exploration of how KHS's 'will to power' actually privileged dying at home as such a positive that clients may find it is difficult to ask for other alternatives. An important research questions would be - Does the discourse of KHS create a feeling of failure in those who cannot cope with looking after their loved ones at home? Does this service give a sense of subtle approval for those who manage their dying in a way deemed appropriate by the positive discourse on 'death with dignity'?

The language/texts suggest that, although the members of KHS support as positive the idea of dying at home, there is a degree of self-reflexivity about this 'good' being interpreted as a 'should'. The following language text suggests the need for further research on this topic by its indication that clients of KHS may feel the pressure of the expectation that a home death is privileged 'both\and' acknowledged by a member of KHS that such an expectation is undesirable.

> We don't in any way pressure...if it seems more appropriate for people to go into an institution then we certainly support them in that and we are

very aware of people feeling, and of people with potential feelings that they have failed or feel guilty and so we do try very hard to avoid that...one women said 'you know I feel really bad because I don't want to die at home and I feel the Karuna nurses will be disappointed'..but we certainly try not to give people that impression (EQ).

This issue needs further research.

The contribution of KHS's spiritual discourse to bioethics

A major contribution of the discourse of KHS, it has been argued, is the *discursive richness of its notion of autonomous choice*. This idea that a discourse (or a different way of talking and acting in regard to end-of-life situations) can make a contribution to bioethics has been used to challenge the more usual *modus operandi* of bioethical reflection - that of Principlism.

In view of such analysis and in consideration of the Nietzschian-cum-Foucaultian notions of the 'will to power' in discourse, the postmodern ethical starting point becomes *not one* of the 'clear and distinct idea'[16] (Jonsen, 1990:Preface) expressed in a well articulated principle, *but rather the discursive support for an interpersonal commitment expressive of a 'will to morality'* (Engelhardt, 1991:120). As Engelhardt proposes (1991:120), it is the desire to engage ethically with fellow humans rather than a clear understanding of foundational assumptions which informs the postmodern language on bioethics. The comfort of totalising reason based on foundational principles is abandoned through the acceptance and challenge of engaging in bioethical reflection in a world of 'moral strangers'[17] where there can be no expectation of communality of moral commitment. As Engelhardt states,

> Though reason fails to discover a content-full *ius naturale* or a common content-full morality for moral strangers, a common morality can come into existence through a common will. It is the will to morality that can set nihilism aside (1991:120).

KHS's spiritual discourse is expressive of such a 'will to morality', as seen by the following comment of a participant,

> (Spirituality) has to do with commitment to be of service to others to be of benefit to others, so that is what I mean by spirituality, it is a genuine wish for giving service to others and not doing for your own ends (EQ).

An important aspect of KHS's contribution to sensitively and constructively handling end-of-life situations rests, it is argued, in the creation and support of their spiritual discourse developed through its clearly articulated and strongly held commitment to be of service to others: in short, its well developed 'will to morality'. Such a will is informed by important notions arising out of the cross- fertilisation of a number of discourses (including the Buddhist, hospice and spiritual discourses). The translation of such 'talk' to action, however, is an extension of the strong commitment, dedication, hard work and inspiration that arises from their 'will to serve'.

The ethical response is not through principles applied to difficult situations, but through a holistic interpretation of the provision of service where the ethical will is expressed throughout the organisational discourse. It is the everyday 'talk' and action of this service that is the *modus operandi* of ethical praxis.

By way of contrast, ethical praxis with regards to end-of-life issues in a tertiary, medical, institutional setting must operate in a number of powerful discourses (the biomedical model, medical professionalism, and economic rationalism), where the everyday 'talk' and action often disempowers and alienates both carer and patient. The application of rational principles in such a situation may be helpful, but does not reach the crux of the problem, which includes issues of discourse power, control and subjectivity.

Recap and summary

The contribution that a study of KHS makes to our understanding and handling of bioethical issues in terminal care is deeper than the application of principles to difficult situations. The discourse of KHS supports an ethical 'will to power' and compassionate subjectivity, which incorporates a holistic view of the individual. Ethical praxis is directed towards empowering the client through the active provision of alternatives and a respect for the individual's right to handle their dying in their own way.

Such a respect begins with an acknowledgment that the service of KHS may not be suitable to everyone, and includes supporting the person to die in their own home (if that is their choice), or referring them to institutional care. The work of members of KHS incorporates a sensitive awareness and response to power issues which arise from the many discourses impacting on the decision making of those facing terminal issues. It is the non-judgmental acceptance and support of the individual in the face of the complexity of these issues of power that IS KHS's different 'way' of responding ethically to end-of-life issues.

Far from being nihilistic, postmodern ideas of discourse and power have been used to suggest an alternative to bioethical reflection which moves the focus away from the more philosophically traditional position of theorising through the application of rational principles, to a concern for the question of the creation of choices. Support for different 'ways' of responding to our terminally ill, it is argued, is as important in seeking bioethical solutions as is the application of principles to the complex and inescapable ethical dilemmas after they arise in a technologically driven, reductionist, medicocentric discourse of today's hi-tech response to dying. Contextualising bioethical problems to issues of power, discourse and the moral 'will' challenges the whole notion of rationalism, because, as Bauman explains,

> ...moral issues cannot be 'resolved', nor the moral life of humanity guaranteed, by the calculating and legislative efforts of reason. Morality is not safe in the hands of reason, though this is exactly what spokesmen of reason promise. Reason cannot help the moral self without depriving the self of what makes the self moral: that unfounded, non-rational, unarguable, no-excuses-give and non-calculable urge to stretch towards the other (1993:247).

Karuna's gift to bioethics is the example they provide by *engaging in their own particular spiritual praxis*.

KHS's contribution to the vexed question of relativism

In concluding this discussion of the relevance of a study of KHS to bioethical reflection will be the suggestion that their discourse goes some way towards demonstrating what shape a postmodern relativist ethical position could take. Such a discussion is not given from a modernist position which seeks progress through the 'once and for all time' resolution of difficult philosophical problems, but rather as comments from the humble findings of local, ad hoc, postmodern research situated in one point in time. Such a postmodern position accepts the irresolvable, paradoxical, aporetic situation ethical theory now confronts. The modest hope is that such findings will contribute some insight into the major crisis which faces ethics (see Chapter 2): and that is making sense of the plurality and incommensurable nature of different ethical world views.

This discussion is informed by two assumptions. Firstly is a respect for Charlesworth's ideal of the liberal democratic society (1994:16) which he states 'is based upon the principle of personal liberty, namely that, to the greatest degree possible, people should be free to make their own life-choices and decisions for themselves...the liberal society is one in which to the maximum degree people are at liberty to exercise their personal autonomy.'

Secondly is Engelhardt's notion that, in the absence of foundational ethical assumptions, the only common ground can be 'the possible bond of mutual respect among persons' (1991:140). Such mutual respect, Engelhardt argues, is the only way of establishing a common moral world without reference to a content-full theory or the ranking of ethical values (1991:119). As our world is full of 'moral strangers', such respect will *ipso facto* necessitate a tolerance of difference. As has been explained previously in this chapter, a presumption of such respect must be the 'will to morality', for without this 'will' there can be no ethical sensibilities. These two assumptions provide the starting point for a postmodern approach to relativism, which privileges desire and difference. What contribution can the discourse of KHS make to understanding these assumptions? Can the 'talk' of KHS provide insights into the ethical challenge of responding to the irreducible pluralistic moralities that exist within our community?

The discourse of KHS shows a high level of self-reflexivity, as demonstrated by the notion that members of this organisation acknowledge that their discourse may not be suitable for everyone. The starting point for their relativism begins at the very boundaries of their discourse. There is no proselytising assumption that others need to, or should, subscribe to their value system. KHS operates on a system of co-opting likeminded individuals into the service and attracting others through their discursive magnet. In short, KHS 'preaches to the converted'. Even at a client level, patients are seen to both self select because of their attraction to Karuna's philosophy, or be selectively referred by health professionals who are sympathetic with the goals of KHS's service. Through an orientation philosophically similar to the Tao of power, members of this organisation 'go with the flow' of the value positions of others respecting not only the right of others to think differently, but also the political inevitability of such difference.

This is contrasted with the many other health organisations that are underpinned by a theologically-driven spirituality (there are many church run hospitals and nursing services) which privileges one particular metaphysical position.

KHS's respect for difference is translated into their everyday work with clients. This is often stressful, demanding work necessitating an ability to work in ambiguous situations. The tension inherent in respect for others can be seen in the following comment by a participant,

> It's a skill I guess of giving them all the options but letting them choose and then feeling alright about that yourself. That's a big thing not to kind of go away feeling you have failed because part of giving people the choice is that that is their choice and they are responsible, you have done the best to support them do what they want to do and that's what you're there for (EQ).

A postmodern orientation to ethics affirms the inevitability of such a tension for, as Bauman explains,

> ...morality is incurably *aporetic*. Few choices (and only those which are relatively trivial and of minor existential importance) are unambiguously good. The majority of moral choices are made between contradictory impulses (1993:11).

This respect for difference partially arises from the Mahayana Buddhist discourse running through this organisation. Such a discourse is known for its tradition of tolerance. As has already been outlined in chapter 5, there are four important notions underpinning this discourse which would affirm such a non-judgmental respect for others. Firstly, this psycho-philosophical view operates on the principle that no one has the right to impose his or her beliefs on another person. Secondly, this is a spiritually-based practice which is more concerned with the engagement in a spiritual journey by demonstrating a caring for others, than it is with philosophical argumentation.[18] Thirdly, the central values are those of compassion (*karuna*) and wisdom (*prajna*) which, when translated into hospice service, create the discursive space for a non-judgmental respect for others. Fourthly, and most importantly, the Mahayana Buddhist tradition asserts a self-reflexive orientation to the construction of reality. Based on the notion of the essential emptiness and relativity of all things, this tradition emphasises the cultivation of an understanding of the construction of the self/no-self (an inward journey), over any notion of changing the 'outside world'. In short, the orientation of such a philosophy is to work with individuals in full acceptance of what they are at that point in time, rather than to impose change from without.

Equally, however, the hospice discourse also supports and affirms this caring, non-judgmental orientation to relating with others. Based on a sensitive appreciation of spirituality as the way the individual makes meaning out of their own life space, the starting point for hospice work is a respect for the meaning-making the individual brings to the dying experience. The hospice experience is about affirming and building on that meaning-making.

Inscribed by many discourses, KHS does not engage in a monotheistic proselytising from any absolutist position, but is actively engaged in a generic spirituality which values a tolerance of a multiplicity of perspectives. As such, KHS's discourse goes some way to incorporating Charlesworth's notion of the liberal, democratic society, and Engelhardt's basic preconditions for ethical engagement in a postmodern world (a respect for others and a 'will to morality'). Such a discourse lends support to Engelhardt's conclusion that,

> In the ruins of modern moral philosophy's hopes, a common morality is still possible. But, moral content must be found amidst the post-modern pluralism of moral visions (1991:140).

Conclusion

Bioethics has been described as 'the disciplined puzzling of people attempting to understand the significance of birth, illness, and death, especially as these are touched on by health care and the biomedical sciences' (Engelhardt, 1986:9). In this chapter, such a 'disciplined puzzling' has attempted to incorporate the insights arising from an exploration of the holistic, spiritual discourse of Karuna Hospice Service.

This understanding has been situated within an awareness of the power of the biomedical discourse and the limits of rationality. The focus of bioethical reflection moved from a concern with the 'clear and distinct idea' expressed in a well articulated principle, to issues of power, discourse, subjectivity and the moral 'will'. In so doing, the foci of ethical praxis became the possibility of discursive support for an interpersonal commitment expressive of a 'will to morality', rather than a concern with formulating rules and general principles.

Within such a theoretical framework, the discursive richness of the KHS notion of autonomous choice was explored and suggested as a constructive 'way' of viewing end-of-life issues. Such a 'way', it was proposed, provided an alternative to the present and dominant bioethical response to ethical dilemmas associated with the dying, which is based in the substantive rationality of Principlism situated in a discourse of technology and medicocentric power. KHS's discourse has been shown to be actively, pragmatically and imaginatively creating the situation in which both the patient and his/her family are supported and provided with choices.

Such a discussion touched on, and included, an exploration of the contribution that such a discourse could make to the present epistemological and metaphysical crises in bioethics: the challenge of making sense of the plurality of incommensurable ethical world views. Discursive notions of tolerance, respect for difference, self-reflexivity, compassion, wisdom, and a practical orientation to spirituality (which is more concerned with engaging in a spiritual journey than intellectual argumentation) went some way to providing insights into a postmodern approach to relativism which incorporated the centrality of desire and difference.

Such a discursive respect of difference and affirmation of the individual's right to choose provided insights into the 'way' the talk of this local, community based hospice engages in protecting and supporting the active, self-determining energy of the individual: referred to in bioethical texts as autonomy. Situated in a spiritual discourse that affirms and respects the importance of meaning making to the individual, such a discursive notion of autonomy is not expressed singularly in the signing of consent forms or the giving of information, but rather incorporates a comprehensive acknowledgment of the significance of the opportunity to choose for individuals.

Throughout this discussion, the focus has remained firmly on the connection between KHS's spiritual discourse and biomedicine. The assumption is that it is at the crossroads of these two discourses that the identity of each is revealed (Rawlinson, 1987:375). As Waitzkin (1989:220) suggests, 'moving beyond the current structure of medical discourse then becomes a major goal of this attempt to analyze it'. In 'moving beyond' the rational approach of biomedicine, an attempt has been made to inscribe in research the value of a spiritual discourse and other ways of knowing for, as Somerville suggests,

> We are not only logical, rational beings, we are also emotional, intuitive, spiritual (which is not the same as religious) ones. Our 'ways of knowing' are complex, diverse and vast (1993:74).

Notes

1 The principle of autonomy has been described by Charlesworth as (1989:70) 'At the most basic level, we have, as human beings, the right to control or determine the course of our own lives and to decide how we shall live (subject of course to our not infringing the rights of others to do the same).'

2 The principle of beneficence demands that 'above all do good'. When applied to a situation this principle requires both the 'provision of benefits'

(preventing and removing harm/doing good) and a 'balancing of benefits and harms' (Johnstone, 1994:93).

3 The next principle, that of non-maleficence, defined as 'above all do no harm' is more clear cut for our society has less an imperative to help than it has a sanction against harming. It is argued that to harm someone is considered morally more indefensible than to refrain from not doing them actual good (Johnstone, 1989:78).

4 Justice has been described by Raphael (1981:68) as 'a complex concept...the most basic of the social virtues and so is in a way the most important of them'. It is too complex to explore in detail in this work.

5 Clouser and Gert (1990:219) referred to this quartet of principles as the 'Georgetown Mantra' because they were originally articulated through the writings of Beauchamp and Childress, academics from Georgetown University and have been so often repeated throughout the bioethical texts that their very names are like a mantra.

6 Interestingly, Nicholson (1994:271) suggests that such an approach to ethics based on a simplistic 'chant' is attractive to physicians who have come through a reductionist memory based medical education system.

7 Holmes (1990:143) expresses this concern well when he writes, 'I contend that the expertise philosophers have in either theoretical or applied ethics does not equip them to make sounder moral judgments on the problems of bioethics than non-philosophers. One cannot "apply" theories like Kantianism or consequentialism to get solutions to practical moral problems unless one knows which theory is correct, and that is a metaethical question over which there is no consensus. On the other hand, to presume to be able to reach solutions through neutral analysis of problems is unavoidably to beg controversial theoretical issues in the process.'

8 Bauman defines 'Aporia' as (1993:8) 'a contradiction that cannot be overcome, one that results in a conflict that cannot be resolved.'

9 Bauman (1993:11) argues that 'moral phenomena are inherently "non-rational". Since they are moral only if they precede the consideration of purpose and the calculation of gains and losses.' In short, there is only a substantive rationality which varies depending on the individual's values and the demands of the situation.

10 Nicholson states (1994:272) 'almost invariably, examples used to discuss the application of the four principles focus attention on a male doctor; rather than questioning the power structure, such examples tend to promote a white, male, western power centre.'

11 There is a strong feminist critique of the use of principlism in ethics as demonstrated by Jaggar's comments (1991:93) that 'even if universal normative principles could be identified, they would have to be given a highly abstract formulation and therefore would necessarily remain vague or indeterminate until they were interpreted in specific contexts...different cultural institutions, and different moral and political practices inevitably would generate different conclusions about right and wrong in specific instances. Unless some universal reason can be identified, there is no way

of choosing some of these interpretations as "correct".'

12 Nicholson writes (1994:271) that 'if anything, however, the intervention of bioethicists has tended to make it easier for doctors and scientists to go ahead with whatever technological innovations they have developed.'

13 Veatch uses the terms medical ethics and bioethics interchangeably, with the suggestion that sometimes bioethics has a slightly broader meaning, including ethical problems of the biological sciences outside medicine (1989:6).

14 The important point of note here is that KHS could offer such choice because its discourse is not based on a biomedical institutional base. The ongoing theme of this research is that, from the very beginning, KHS did not have a medicocentric discourse. This is an important consideration in regards to understanding the possibility of this service creating a different 'way' of responding to the dying. As Russell (1989:23) records, research on hospice organisations suggests that those originally associated with preexisting medical institutions 'tend to be characterised by processes that counteract change, thus maintaining the status quo'. The 'linchpin' or key figure to starting this service was a Buddhist monk with a professional background in physiotherapy. This is not only an important factor in understanding the following contribution to bioethical reflection, but an indication of the possible difficulty of reproducing this service elsewhere. The assumption is not made that there are a preponderance of Buddhist monks with physiotherapy degrees who have the charisma and driving commitment to develop a community based hospice. This leadership along with the many other factors contributing to making this service different (as outlined in Chapter 5) may or may not be duplicated elsewhere. Certainly, however, the hospice literature worldwide indicates the possibility of similar but different successful attempts at humanising the experience of dying. Whilst stressing the theoretical limitations, however, it is the author's hope that the voice of experience of those engaged in forming this service may make some contribution to the development of such services elsewhere.

15 The bioethicists Pellegrino and Thomasma (1988:3) trace the philosophical notions of liberty and autonomy of the individual to the Enlightenment (French and English) where they argue that it gathered strength during the nineteenth century in response to the depreciation of personal worth that accompanied the Industrial Revolution.

16 Engelhardt (1991:xiii) defines 'moral strangers' as 'the relationship people have to one another when they are involved in moral controversies and do not share a concrete moral vision that provides the basis for the resolution of controversies, but instead regard one another as acting out of fundamentally divergent moral commitments.'

17 As Jonsen (1990: Preface) explains, Descartes was the archmentor of rationality, whose ontological premise 'cognito ergo sum', championed the 'clear and distinct idea' as the ideal underpinning ethical reasoning.

18 This is a particularly poignant point when placed in the context of the central concern of this chapter, and that is the limits of the approach to

bioethics of rationalistic principlism. Holmes (1990:157) from within the literature of bioethics articulates a similar point when he poses the question of 'what relevance does philosophical ethics have to solving the problems of bioethics? Some, I suggest, but not much..The cultivation of a morally sensitive, caring, and compassionate character probably counts for more in the end than any analytical skills.'

14 A concluding statement

> We shall not cease from exploration
> And the end of all our exploring
> Will be to arrive where we started
> And know the place for the first time
> (Eliot cited in Grof and Grof, 1989:191).

To return to the myth of Daedalus, this work seeks to affirm the significance of the notion of a spiritual discourse as a 'way' of responding to the bioethical dilemmas associated with the recent, extensive and intrusive use of technology in the care of the dying. The conclusion is that a different (spiritual) 'way' of thinking about and talking about death and dying, does, indeed, directly and actively translate into a different construction of 'reality' for the care of the terminally ill.

In view of the dearth of research on spirituality and the previously documented (Chapter 2) difficulties encountered by modernist epistemological approaches for exploring the notion of a transcendent dimension, the documentation of such findings on spirituality is considered important.

Spirituality and research: creating the link

Spirituality, dubbed the 'ignored dimension' (Soeken and Carson, 1986:52), has received scant research attention (Chapman, 1986:41; Ross, 1994:441; Soeken and Carson, 1986:52; Forbes, 1994:297; Stiles, 1990:236; Kaye and Robinson, 1994:219). This paucity of research exists in spite of the expressed understanding that illness and suffering are by their very nature spiritual encounters (Belcher, Dettmore, and Holzemer, 1989:16). The research that does exist suggests that during times of illness and crises (such as dying) spiritual issues become more important to the individual (Emblem and

Halstead, 1993:176), and the search for meaning becomes even more intensified (Sims, 1987:63). Understandably, as Stepnick and Perry point out (1992:17), such a dearth of research on the notion of spirituality is 'particularly unjustifiable when the client is terminally ill and approaching death'.

It has been a recurring theme of this work that modern western responses to terminal illness are based on a reductionist, scientific understanding of biomedicine. Scientific epistemologies underpin our modernist ways of knowing about the dying experience. Even where such knowledge includes a psycho-social dimension, it is still underpinned by science, because, historically, behavioural and social 'scientists' adopted their model of research from the physical sciences (Fahlberg and Fahlberg, 1991:276). The danger is as Diaz explains, that these naturalistic methodologies 'often place an arbitrary restriction on knowing anything outside of that which is attainable through scientific methodology' (1993:325). The 'murky and uncomfortable esoteric nature' of the notion of spirituality (Chapman, 1986:39) would be and is, a dimension easily marginalised by the methodological hegemony of scientism and naturalism.[1] The chief obstacle to progress in this area is the difficulty associated with trying to scientifically measure the human spiritual nature (Bensley, 1991:353). The problem becomes as Fahlberg and Fahlberg suggest,

> If spirituality is a part of human experience, then we seem to need an expanded science, or at least an expanded epistemology to study spirituality - not only directly but also in terms of its empirical and rational manifestations. Human science, the consciousness disciplines, and the willingness to make forays into the unknown may be essential resources in this quest (1991:280).

This work not only affirms the importance and relevance of the notion of spirituality, (in this case in relation to the 'difference' and 'resistance' of a Buddhist based community hospice) but also sought to demonstrate the use of a postmodern research framework as one such possibility of Fahlberg and Fahlberg's notion of an 'expanded epistemology'. It is one of the conclusions reached, that the use of postmodern ideas of discourse have been most productive for making such 'forays into the unknown'.

By challenging the notion of rationalism and situating this research in postmodern notions of discourse and power, an important outcome has been to show that for those associated with the work of Karuna Hospice Service the notion of spirituality is in an active relationship to the construction of reality for both worker and client. The implication of this spiritual 'talk' has been explored at both the organisational level and at the coalface of patient care. As this is postmodern research which does not seek to prove, quantify or establish the 'truth' of such a notion,[2] this construction of reality has been acknowledged, affirmed, and recorded.

Thus, by using the perspective of postmodern epistemological assumptions, the notion of spirituality has been made examinable and discussable through discourse. Through discourse the notion of spirituality is identifiable, and through a postmodern epistemological framework, such identifiable 'talk' is made available for research. In short, a postmodern focus on discourse provides one way of accessing the notion of spirituality as 'data' for research. Articulating such a process is seen as one contribution of this work.

From data to interpretation

While positivist research would be informed by a notion of a 'non-situated, disembedded, disinterested person' who is creator or author of the work, a postmodern approach 'accepts that there are no ideal observers who can be abstracted from their social situation' (Davis, 1995:27). Each piece of research will be situated in and depend on the researcher(s)'s *'aesthetics of existence'*.[3]

As *part of the KHS discursive magnet*, I have been attracted to this organisation's democratic and holistic vision. My experiences have been invariably positive and have affirmed all that I have been told.[4] Experientially and philosophically, my involvement has resonated with and affirmed the many notions that have emerged and been inscribed in this research. This does not mean *ipso facto* that such values were directly and simply translated into the interpretation or that what was hoped to be found was indeed, found. My interpretations are dependent on the data collected, which is available for further interpretation, situated intertextually in the literature on this topic, and subject to innumerable readings by others in the production of the final text.[5] Such values did, however, have a powerful impact directly on the construction of this text.

The interesting point which emerged (for myself) from this sojourn into postmodern literature, is that whilst a multiplicity of possible readings is acknowledged and valued, indeed invited, there is not a concomitant responsibility to incorporate such readings in the construction of one's own text. The original fear that a nihilist denial of any position was the *sine qua non* of the postmodern approach, has (in the author's experience) been challenged by the actual doing of this research. Writing, the inscription of ideas in words, is the actual taking of a position. Even a nihilist choosing not to take a position is still taking a position.

To pen one's beliefs in words, is, *ipso facto,* to epistemologically and psychologically to believe those statements to be true. The modernist position would be to accept this truth as absolute. Postmodern writers accept the tension (Postmodern Irony) of making statements of belief whilst always aware that such a position is contingent and subject to change (Rorty, 1989:73-4).

Future inquiry

Already within this text are the future seeds of deconstruction suggested by the need for further research. Rather than seek closure, the interpretation of data has been made in a spirit of openness and a valuing of uncertainty. At many points in the development of ideas, such inconclusiveness did not justify grand leaps of theoretical faith, but rather suggested the need for further research. This need for further research has been acknowledged at appropriate points throughout this text.

The outcome of such research would further inform (and deconstruct) the present interpretation of findings as can be seen by the following suggested list of questions:

- Does the KHS discourse put pressure on clients to show they can cope with (or desire) a home death?
- Does a discourse on spirituality marginalise the useful expression of individual needs and wants?
- Is there more conflict and fallout during the formative stage of a project than there is during the period of routinization?
- Does a shared spiritual framework foster or hinder the expression and resolution of more destructive human dynamics?
- Can the contrast between the early conflict and the present contentment suggest an evolutionary and positive operation of a spiritual discourse?
- Why was the notion of *karma*, a central Buddhist concept, not mentioned during the interviews?
- Is KHS's Taoist philosophy only effective for providing for those in the system who are already able to provide for themselves?
- How inclusive is the clientele of KHS in terms of a social justice agenda which responds to a wide variety of marginalised and disempowered individuals?
- What is the impact of perfectionism on this service and what is the support for establishing worker boundaries on what they are prepared to do?
- Is Cittimani (the alternative KHS hospice run purely on a voluntary base on the sunshine coast) different in anyway from the Brisbane service?
- Is it significant that the idea of euthanasia was not mention by those interviewed, and if so, what are the implications of this silence?

Concluding the conclusion

The serious intent behind this research has been a desire to engage in the ethical praxis of constructing different ways of seeing (a postmodern approach to research) which may go some way in protecting more marginalised ways of knowing (spiritual and hospice) from the hegemony of powerful discourses (positivism and biomedicine). In doing so I have managed to inscribe one view of KHS's 'reality' and this view has managed to inscribe something of me. For as Davis (1993) suggests,

> I am a snail that carries my home with me on the journey. I cannot separate the 'me' from the 'journey' in the same way that I cannot separate my epistemology from my ontology or my ethic from my self identity and world view.

Such a world view is humbled, touched and inspired by a group of people who can so energetically and caringly translate their vision into a 'reality' which can embrace others at perhaps the most vulnerable and challenging time of their existence.

'May a thousand Karunas blossom'

Notes

1 According to Casti (1989) the implicit assumption in scientism becomes 'science = truth'. As Fahlberg and Fahlberg explains, 'most scientists, then, advocated the material notion of science exclusively, and they gradually became unable to distinguish science from scientism...the doctrine of scientism holds that what does not exist materially, does not exist at all' (1991:276). Spirituality by its very esoteric nature is obviously marginalised or eliminated in such a way of knowing.

2 This is not to deny that many scientific researchers, particularly physicists, are interested in exploring the possibility of establishing an interrelationship between empirical reality and a transcendent understanding of the universe. There is a recent and explicitly stated interest in the connection between 'science and the search for ultimate meaning' (Davies, 1992), (Davies, 1983; Hawking, 1962; Heisenberg, 1962; Smoot and Davidson, 1993; Koestler, 1976; Capra, 1991; Capra and Steindl-Rast, 1992; Dyson, 1988; de Duve, 1995).

3 Patton (1986:138) uses the term 'aesthetic of existence' to refer to the postmodern epistemological notion that the individual's subjectivity is formed by power, discourse and desire. Patton, consequently argues for the possibility of 'an ethic which judges practices not by reference to a universal moral code but to an aesthetic of existence'.

4 This has included experiences with the perceived negative aspects of perfectionism and relationships with those hurt and marginalised by this service.

5 This research was completed as doctoral research and hence was subjected to the scrutiny of university supervision and examination.

Bibliography

Aaron, H. and Schwartz, W., (1984) *The Painful Prescription: Rationing Hospital Care,* The Brooking Institution, Washington, D.C.

Aaron, H. and Schwartz, W., (1985) "Hospital Cost Control: A Bitter Pill to Swallow", *Harvard Business Review,* March/April: 160-161.

Abel, E., (1986) "The Hospice Movement: Institutionalizing Innovation",*International Journal of Health Services,* 16,1:71-85.

Albrecht, G. and Higgins, P., (1979) *Health, Illness and Medicine,* Rand McNally, Chicago.

Alderson, P., (1991) "Abstract Bioethics Ignores Human Emotions", *Bulletin of Medical Ethics,* May:13-21.

Almond, B., (1988) "Philosophy, Medicine and its Technologies", *Journal of Medical Ethics,* 14:173-178.

Andrews, L., (1986) "My Body, My Property", *Hastings Center Report,* 16:28-38.

Annas, G., (1991) "The Health Care Proxy and the Living Will", *The New England Journal of Medicine,* 324:1210-1213.

Anspach, R., (1990) "The Language of Case Presentation", in *Sociology of Health and Illness: Critical Perspectives,* Conrad, P. and Kern, R., (eds)., St Martin's Press, New York.

Arac, J., (ed.), (1990) *Postmodernism and Politics,* University of Minnesota Press, Minneapolis.

Aries, P., (1991) *The Hour of Our Death,* Oxford University Press, Oxford.

Armstrong, D., (1987) "Theoretical Tensions in Biopsychosocial Medicine", *Social Science and Medicine,* 25,11:1213-1218.

Arney, R. and Bergen, B., (1983) "The Anomaly, the Chronic Patient and the Play of Medical Power", *Sociology of Health and Illness,* 5,1:1-24.

Aronowitz, S., (1992) "The Tensions of Critical Theory: Is Negative Dialectics All There Is?", in *Postmodernism & Social Theory,* Seidman, S. and Agner, D., (eds.), Basil Blackwell, Cambridge.Atkins, G., (1983) *Reading*

Deconstruction, Deconstruction Reading, The University Press of Kentucky, Kentucky.

Auer, J., (1990) "Psychological Problems in Chronic Illness", in *Social Work Practice in Health Care,* Badawi, M. and Biamonti, B., (eds.), Woodhead-Faulkner, New York.

Bailey, S., (1996) "Levels of Empathy of Critical Care Nurses", *Australian Critical Care,* 9,4:121-127.

Baillie, L., (1996) "A Phenomenological Study of the Nature of Empathy", *Journal of Advanced Nursing,* 24:1300-1308.

Banks, R., (1980) "Health and the Spiritual Dimension: Relationskhips and Implications for Professional Preparation Programs", *Journal of School Health,* 50,4:195-202.

Barnard, D., (1988) "Love and Death: Existential Dimensions of Physicians' Difficulties with Moral Problems", *The Journal of Medicine and Philosophy,* 13:393-409.

Barrett, M., (1991) *The Politics of Truth: From Marx to Foucault,* Polity Press, Cambridge.

Bass, D., (1985) "The Hospice Ideology and Success of Hospice Care", *Research on Aging,* 7, 3:307-327.

Batchelor, S., (1990) "Mahayana Spirituality", in *Space in Mind,* Crook, J. and Fontana, D., (eds.), Element Books, London.

Bates, E. and Birch, C., (1981) *Science and Ethics, Part 2, The Human Cost of Medical Technology,* Australian Broadcasting Commission, (sound recording).

Bates, E. and Lapsley, H., (1985) *The Health Machine: The Impact of Medical Technology,* Penguin, Victoria.

Bates, E. and Linder-Pelz, S., (1987) *Health Care Issues,* Allen and Unwin, Sydney.

Bauman, Z., (1988) "Is There a Postmodern Sociology?", *Theory, Culture and Society,* 5,2-3:217-238.

Bauman, Z., (1993) *Postmodern Ethics,* Blackwell, Oxford.

Bayer, R., Callahan, D., Fletcher, J., Hodgson, T., Jennings, B., Monsees, D., Sieverts, S. and Veatch, R., (1983) "The care of the Terminally Ill: Morality and Economics", *The New England of Medicine,* 309,24:1490-1494.

Bayertz, K., (1992) "Techno-Thanatology: Moral consequences of Introducing Brain Criteria for Death", *Journal of Medicine and Philosophy,* 17:407-417.

Beardsley, T., (1994) "A War Not Won", *Scientific American,* January:118-126.

Beauchamp, T. and Childress, J., (1983) *Principles of Biomedical Ethics,* 2nd Edition, Oxford University Press, Oxford.

Beauchamp, T. and Walters, L., (1982) *Contemporary Issues in Bioethics,* 3rd Edition, Wadsworthy Publishing, California.

Becker, E., (1973) *The Denial of Death,* The Free Press, New York.

Bedell, S., Delbanco, T.,Cook, F. and Epstein, F., (1983) "Survival After Cardiopulmonary Resuscitation in the Hospital", *The New England Journal of Medicine,* 309,10:569-576.

Bedell, S. and Delbanco, T., (1986) "Choices About Cardiopulmonary Resuscitation in the Hospital", *The New England Journal of Medicine,* 310:1089-1093.
Behavioural and Social Sciences Ethical Review Committee, (BSSERC) (1992) *Procedures and Guidelines for Ethical Review,* University of Queensland.
Belcher, A., Dettmore, D. and Holzemer, S., (1989) "Spirituality and Sense of Well-being in Persons with AIDS", *Holistic Nursing Practice,* 3,4:16-25.
Bellingham, R., Cohen, B., Jones, T. and Spaniol, L., (1989) "Connectedness: Some Skills for Spiritual Health", *American Journal of Health Promotion,* 4,1:18-31.
Bendix, R., (1966) *Max Weber,* Methuen, London.
Bennett, J., (1995) "Methodological Notes on Empathy", *Advanced Nursing Science,* 18,1:36-50.
Bensley, R., (1991) "Spiritual Health as a Component of Worksite Health Promotion/Wellness Programming: A Review of the Literature", *Journal of Health Education,* Nov/Dec.,22,6:352-394.
Berger, P. and Luckmann, T., (1966) *The Social Construction of Reality,* Penguin Books, England.
Berliner, H., (1984) "Scientific Medicine Since Flexner", *Alternative Medicines, Popular and Policy Perspectives,* (ed.), Salmon, J., Tavistock, London.
Best, J., (1987) "High Technology - The Problems of Progress", *The Medical Journal of Australia,* 146,16/2:220-223.
Best, S. and Kellner, K., (1991) *Postmodern Theory, Critical Interrogations,* Macmillan, London.
Bird, O., (1976) *Cultures in Conflict: An Essay in the Philosophy of the Humanities,* University of Notre Dame Press, Notre Dame.
Black, D., (1988) *Health at the Crossroads,* Tapestry Press, Australia.
Blackhall, L., (1987) "Sounding Board : Must We Always Use CPR?", *The New England Journal of Medicine,* 317,20:1281-1285.
Blues, A. and Zerwekh, J., (1984) *Hospice and Palliative Nursing Care,* Grune and Stratton, London.
Blum, F., (1970) "Getting Individuals to Give Information to the Outsider" in *Qualitative Methodology,* Filstead, W., (ed.), Markman Publishing Company, Chicago.
Blum, L., (1980) *Friendship, Altruism and Morality,*Routledge and Kegan Paul, London.
Boisaubin, E., (1993) "Legal Decisions Affecting the Limitation of Nutritional Support", *The Hospice Journal,* 9,(2/3):131-147.
Bok, S., (1976) "Personal Directions for Care at the End of Life", *The New England Journal of Medicine,* 295,7:367-369.
Bolton, R., (1987) *People Skills: How to Assert Yourself, Listen to Others, and Resolve Conflicts,* Simon and Schuster, Brookvale.
Borges, S., (1986) "A Feminist Critique of Scientific Ideology: An Analysis of Two Doctor-Patient Encounters", in *Discourse and Institutional Authority: Medicine, Education and Law,* Fisher, S. and Todd, A., (eds.), Vol xix, Alex

Publishing Co., Norwood.
Boyle, J., (1984) "Should We Learn to Say No?", *Journal of American Medical Association,* 252:782-84.
Boyne, R. and Rattansi, A., (1990) *Postmodernism and Society,* Macmillan, London.
Bransen, E., (1992) "Has Menstruation Been Medicalised? Or Will it Never Happen...", *Sociology of Health and Illness,* 14,1:98-110.
Breindel, C. and Boyle, R., (1979) "Implementing a Multiphased Hospice Program", *Hospital Progress,* 3:42-45.
Britten, N., (1991) "Hospital Consultants' Views of Their Patients", *Sociology of Health and Illness,* 13,1:83-97.
Brock, D., (1989) "Death and Dying" in *Medical Ethics,* Veatch, R., (ed.), Jones and Bartlett Publishers, Boston.
Brody, H., (1987) "Cost Containment as Professional Challenge", *Theoretical Medicine,* 8:5-17.
Brody, H., (1989) "The Physician/Patient Relationship", in *Medical Ethics,* Veatch, R., (ed.), Jones and Bartlett Publishers, Boston.
Brooke, V., (1987) "The Spiritual Well-Being of the Elderly", *Geriatric Nursing,* July/August:194-195.
Brubaker, R., (1984) *The Limits of Rationality: An Essay on the Social and Moral Thought of Max Weber,* George Allen and Unwin, London.
Burgess, R., (1982) "The Unstructured Interview as a Conversation", in *Field Research: A Sourcebook & Field Manual,* Burgess, R., (ed.), George Allen & Unwin, London.
Burnard, P., (1988) "Searching For Meaning", *Nursing Times,* September 14,84,37:34-36.
Bury, M., (1986) "Social Constructionism and the Development of Medical Sociology", *Sociology of Health and Illness,* 8:137-169.
Byrd, S. and Taylor, K., (1989) "Evaluating a Hospice Program: A Practical Approach", *American Journal of Hospice Care,* 6,1:41-46.
Cairns, J., (1978) *Cancer: Science and Society,* Freeman and Co., San Francisco.
Callahan, D., (1993) "Pursuing a Peaceful Death", *Hastings Center Report,* July-August:33-38.
Callahan, D., (1994) "Bioethics: Private Choice and Common Good", *Hastings Center Report,* May-June:28-31.
Callahan, J., (ed.), (1988) *Ethical Issues in Professional Life,* Oxford University Press, Oxford.
Calnan, M. and Williams, S., (1992) "Images of Scientific Medicine",*Sociology of Health and Illness,* 14,2:233-254.
Campbell, A., Gillett, G. and Jones, G., (1992) *Practical Medical Ethics,* Oxford University Press, Melbourne.
Campbell, J., (1988) *The Power of Myth,* Doubleday, New York.
Campbell, K., (1970) *Body and Mind,* Macmillan, London.
Capra, F., (1990) *The Turning Point : Science, Society and the Rising Culture,* Flamingo Books, London.
Capra, F., (1991) *The Tao of Physics,* Shambhala, Boston.

Capra, F. and Steindl-Rast,D., (1992) *Belonging to the Universe,* Penguin Books, London.
Card, C., (ed.), (1991) *Feminist Ethics,* University of Kansas, Kansas.
Card, C., (1991) "The Feistiness of Feminism", in *Feminist Ethics,* Card, C., (ed.), University of Kansas, Kansas.
Carson, R., (1994) "Sensiblility and Rationality in Bioethics", *Hastings Center Report,* May-June:23-24.
Carr-Gregg, M. and Hobbs, K., (1988) "The Technological Imperative and Institutional Abuse: Its Effect on the Young Person with Cancer", *Australian Social Work,* June,41,2:25-29.
Cassell, E., (1991a) *The Nature of Suffering and the Goals of Medicine,*Oxford University Press, Oxford.
Cassell, E., (1991b) "Recognizing Suffering", *Hastings Center Report,*May/June:24-31.
Cassell, E., (1993) "The Sorcerer's Broom: Medicine's Rampant Technology", *Hastings Center Report,* November-December:32-39.
Cassidy, S., (1991) *Sharing the Darkness: The Spirituality of Caring,* Orbis Books, New York.
Casti, J., (1989) *Paradigms Lost,* Avon Books, New York, NY.
Chalmers, A., (1976) *What is This Thing Called Science,* University of Queensland Press, Brisbane.
Chapman, L., (1986) "Spiritual Health: A Component Missing From Health Promotion", *American Journal of Health Promotion,* 1,1:38-41.
Charlesworth, M., (1989) *Life, Death, Genes and Ethics,* Boyer Lectures, Australian Broadcasting Commission Book, Crows Nest.
Charlesworth, M., (1993) *Bioethics in a Liberal Society,* Cambridge University Press, Melbourne.
Charnes, L. and Moore, P., (1992) "Meeting Patients' Spiritual Needs: The Jewish Perspective", *Holistic Nursing Practice,* 6,3:64-72.
Chau, T., (1991) "Five Principles for a New Global Moral Order", in *Buddhism and Nonviolent Global Problem-solving,* Paige, G. and Gilliatt, S., (eds.), Center for Global Nonviolence Planning Project, Spark Matsunaga Institute for Peace, University of Hawaii, Honolulu.
Cheek, J. and Rudge, T., (1993) "The Power of Normalisation: Foucauldian Perspectives on Contemporary Australian Health Care Practices", *Social Issues,* 28,4:271-284.
Cheek, J. and Rudge, T., (1994) "Webs of Documentation: The Discourse of Case Notes", *Australian Journal of Communication,* 21,2:41-51.
Ch'en, K., (1968) *Buddhism, The Light of Asia,* Barron's Educational Series, New York.
Cherry, L., (1982) "Hospices: New Help for the Dying", *Glamour,* March:256-314.
Chervenak, F. and McCullough, L., (1991) "Justifying Limits on Refusing Intervention", *Hastings Center Report,* March/April:12-18.
Clark, C., Cross, J., Deane, K. and Lowry, L., (1991) "Spirituality: Integral to Quality Care", *Holistic Nursing Practice,* 5,3,:67-76.
Clark, D., (ed.), (1993) *The Future of Palliative Care: Issues of Policy and*

Practice, Open University Press, Buckingham.
Clark, D., (1993) "Wither the Hospices?", in *The Future of Palliative Care: Issues of Policy and Practice,* Open University Press, Buckingham.
Clark, J. and Mishler, E., (1992) "Attending to Patients' Stories: Reframing the Clinical Task", *Sociology of Health and Illness,* 14,3:344-372.
Clooney, F., (1995) "Back to the Basics: Reflections on Moral Discourse in a Contemporary Hindu Community", *The Journal of Medicine and Philosophy,* 20:439-457.
Clouser, K. and Gert, B., (1990) "A Critique of Principlism", *The Journal of Medicine and Philosophy,* 15:219-236.
Cochrane, J., Levy, M. and Oglesby, C., (1990-91) "Death Anxiety, Disclosure Behaviours, and Attitudes of Oncologists Toward Terminal Care", *Omega,* 22,1:1-12.
Comaroff, J., (1982) "Medicine: Symbol and Ideology", in *The Problem of Medical Knowledge,* Wright, P. and Treacher, A., Edinburgh University Press, Edinburgh.
Coney, S., (1988) *The Unfortunate Experiment,* Penguin Books, Auckland.
Corbett, T. and Hai, D., (1979) "Searching for Euthanatos: The Hospice Alternative", *Hospital Progress,* 60:38-41.
Corr, C. and Corr, D., (1983) *Hospice Care: Principles and Practice,* Faber and Faber, London.
Courtenay, B., (1993) *April Fool's Day,* William Heinemann Australia, Victoria.
Crawshaw, R., (1983) "Technical Zeal or Therapeutic Purpose - How to Decide?", *Journal of American Medical Association,* 250,14:1857-59.
Creek, L., (1982) "A Homecare Hospice Profile: Description, Evaluation, and Cost Analysis", *The Journal of Family Practice,* 14,1:53-58.
Crook, J., (1990) "East-West Psychology: Towards a Meeting of Minds", in *Space in Mind, Crook,* Crook, J. and Fontana, D., (eds.), Element Books, London.
Crook, J. and Fontana, D., (eds.), (1990) *Space in Mind,* Element Books, London.
Crowther, C., (1980) "The Stalled Hospice Movement", *New Physician,*29:26-28.
Darragh, W., (1994) "Loving Jordan", *The Karuna Hospice News,* December:1-2.
Dalai Lama, The, (1995) *The Power of Compassion,* Thorsons, Glasgow.
Daly, J., (1989) "Innocent Murmurs: Echocardiography and the Diagnosis of Cardiac Normality", *Sociology of Health and Illness,* 11,2:99-116.
Davies, B., (1994) *Poststructuralist Theory and Classroom Practice,* Deakin University, Geelong.
Davies, P., (1983) *God and The New Physics,* Penguin, London.
Davies, P., (1992) *The Mind of God, Science and the Search for Ultimate Meaning,* Penguin Books, London.
Davion, V., (1991) "Integrity and Social Change" in *Feminist Ethics,* Card, C., (ed.), University Press of Kansas, Lawerence.
Davis, K., (1993) "Who are We Kidding, Action Research for Whom?", in

Critical Theory Feminism and Nursing, Empowering Nursing's Future, National Nursing Conference, Proceedings, Quality Health Forums, Melbourne.
Davis, K., (1995) "Avoiding Discrepancy Between Moral Theory and Social Reality in the Context of Health Research", *Autonomy, Community and Justice in Bioethics,* Proceedings, University of Queensland Press, Brisbane.
Dear, M., (1988) "The Postmodern Challenge: Reconstructing Human Geography", *Trans Institute British Geography,* 13:262-274.
de Duve, C., (1995) "Life and Meaning in the Universe", *The Futurist,* May-June:60.
Degner, L., Gow, C. and Thompson, L., (1991) "Critical Nursing Behaviors in Care for the Dying", *Cancer Nursing,* 14,5:246-253.
Degrazia, D., (1992) "Moving Forward in Bioethical Theory: Theories, Cases and Specified Principlism", *The Journal of Medicine and Philosophy,* 17:511-539.
Dellaport, W., (1987) "Paediatric Update : Children Who Have had Cancer, Did We Really Cure Them?", *Cancer Nursing,* 10, (Suppl. 1):115-120.
Devereux, J., Jones, D. and Dickenson, D., (1993) "Can Children Withhold Consent to Treatment?", *British Medical Journal,* 306:1459-1461.
Diaz, D., (1993) "Foundations for Spirituality: establishing the Viability of Spirituality Within the Health Disciplines", *Journal of Health Education,* Nov/Dec.,24,6:324-326.
Dobratz, M., (1990) "Hospice Nursing: Present Perspectives and Future Directives", *Cancer Nursing,* 13,2:116-122.
Docherty, T., (1990) *After Theory, Postmodernism/Postmarxism,* Routledge, London.
Doherty, R., (Chairman), (1980) *The New Curriculum - Medicine 1, 1979,* Report to the Faculty of Medicine by the Curriculum Evaluation Sub-Committee, University of Queensland, Brisbane.
Donchin, A., (1989) "The Growing Feminist Debate Over the New Reproductive Technologies", *Hypatia,* 4,3:136-149.
Douglas, M., (1986) "The Social Preconditions of Radical Scepticism", in *Power, Action and Belief,* Law, J., (ed.), Routledge, London.
Downie, R. and Calman, K., (1987) *Healthy Respect: Ethics in Health Care,* Faber and Faber, London.
Doyle, D., (1979) *Terminal Care,* Churchill Livingstone, Edinburgh.
Doyle, D., Hanks, G. and Macdonald, N., (1993) *Oxford Textbook of Palliative Medicine,* Oxford University Press, Oxford.
DuBois, P., (1980) *The Hospice Way of Death,* Human Science Press, New York.
Dunstan, G. and Shinebourne, E., (eds.), (1989) *Doctors' Decisions: Ethical Conflicts in Medical Practice,* Oxford University Press, Oxford.
Dush, D., (1988) "Psychological Research in Hospice Care: Toward Specificity of Therapeutic Mechanisms", *The Hospice Journal,* 4,2:9-36.
Dush, D., (1988) "Trends in Hospice Research and Psychosocial Palliative Care", *The Hospice Journal,* 4,3:13-29.
Dutton, D., (1988) *Worse Than The Disease: Pitfalls of Medical Progress,*

Cambridge University Press, Cambridge.
Dworkin, G., (1988) *The Theory and Practice of Autonomy*, Cambridge University Press, Cambridge.
Dyson, F., (1988) *Infinite in All Directions*, Penguin Books, London.
Eco, U., (1989) *Foucault's Pendulum*, Secker and Warburg, London.
Edwards, M. and Tolle, S., (1993) "Disconnecting a Ventilator at the Request of a Patient Who Knows He Will Then Die: The Doctor's Anguish", *Annals of Internal Medicine*, 117,3:254-256.
Ehrenreich, J., (1978) *The Cultural Crisis of Modern Medicine*, Monthly Review Press, New York.
Elam, D., (1994) *Feminism and Deconstruction*, Routledge, New York.
Ellard, J., (1991) "On the Distribution of Resources", *Modern Medicine of Australia*, 6/12:24-29.
Emblen, J. and Halstead, L., (1993) "Spiritual Needs and Interventions: Comparing the Views of Patients, Nurses, and Chaplains" *Clinical Nurse Specialist*, 7,4:175-182.
Emblen, J., (1992) "Religion and Spirituality Defined According to Current Use in Nursing Literature", *Journal of Professional Nursing*, 8,1:41-47.
Emanuel, E., (1995) "The Beginning of the End of Principlism", *Hastings Center Report*, July-August:37-38.
Emanuel, L., (1991) "PSDA in the Clinic", *Hastings Center Report, Special Supplement*, September-October:S6-S7.
Emanuel, L., Barry, M., Stoeckle, J., Ettelson, L. and Emanuel, E., (1991) "Advance Directives for Medical Care- A Case for Greater Use", *Bioethics News*, 11,1:20-33.
Engelhardt, H., (1986) *The Foundations of Bioethics*, Oxford University Press, Oxford.
Engelhardt, H., (1991) *Bioethics and Secular Humanism: The Search for a Common Morality*, Trinity Press International, Philadelphia.
Engelhardt, H. and Wildes, K., (1994) "The Four Principles of Health Care Ethics and Post-modernity: Why a Libertarian Interpretation is Unavoidable", in *Principles of Health Care Ethics*, Gillon, R., (ed.), John Wiley and Sons, Chichester.
Evans, A. and Brody, D., (1985) "The Do-Not-Resuscitate Order in Teaching Hospitals", *Journal of American Medical Association*, 253:2236-2239.
Evatt, P., (1995) *Needs Analysis of Training in Palliative Care for Health Professionals*, Masters Thesis, University of Queensland, Brisbane.
Fahlberg, L. and Fahlberg, L., (1991) "Exploring Spirituality and Consciousness with and Expanded Science: Beyond the Ego with Empiricism, Phenomenology, and Contemplation", *American Journal of Health Promotion*, 5,4:273-281.
Fairclough, N., (1985) "Critical and Descriptive Goals in Discourse Analysis", *Journal of Pragmatics*, 9:739-763.
Fairclough, N., (1989) *Language and Power*, Longman, London.
Fairclough, N., (1992) *Discourse and Social Change*, Polity Press, Cambridge.
Fairman, J., (1992) "Watchful Vigilance: Nursing Care, Technology, and the Development of Intensive Care Units", *Nursing Research*, Jan/Feb,40,1:56-

59.
Farrell, J., (1982) "The Dying of Death: Historical Perspectives", *Death Education,* 6:105-123.
Faulder, C., (1985) *Whose Body is it? The Troubling Issue of Informed Consent,* Virago, Bristol.
Fay, B., (1975) *Social Theory and Political Practice,* George Allen and Unwin, Boston.
Fay, B., (1987) *Critical Social Science: Liberation and Its Limits,* Cornell University Press, New York.
Featherstone, M., (1988) "In Pursuit of Postmodern: An Introduction", *Theory, Culture and Society,* 5,2-3:195-216.
Fernando, A., (1985) *Buddhism Made Plain,* Orbis Books, New York.
Field, D. and James, N., (1993) "Where and How People Die", in *The Future of Palliative Care,* Clark, D., (ed.), Open University Press, Buckingham.
Fife, B., (1994) "The Conceptualization of Meaning in Illness", *Social Science and Medicine,* 38,2:309-316.
Filstead, W., (ed.), (1970) *Qualitative Methodology,* Markham Publishing Company, Chicago.
Finkler, K., (1991) *Physicians at Work, Patients in Pain: Biomedical Practice and Patient Response in Mexico,* Westview Press, Oxford.
Finnis, J., (1993) "Withdrawing Nutrition and Hydration", *Bioethics Outlook,* 4,3:1-2.
Fisher, M. and Raper, R., (1990) "Withdrawing and Withholding Treatment in Intensive Care", *The Medical Journal of Australia,* 153,20/8:217-224.
Fisher, S., (1991) "A Discourse of the Social: Medical Talk/Power Talk/Oppositional Talk?", *Discourse and Society,* 2,2:157-182.
Fisher, S. and Todd, A., (1986a) "Introduction: Communication in Institutional Contexts: Social Interaction and Social Structure", in *Discourse and Institutional Authority: Medicine, Education and Law,* Fisher, S. and Todd, A., (eds.), Vol. xix, Alex Publishing Co., Norwood.
Fisher, S. and Todd, A., (1986b) *Discourse and Institutional Authority: Medicine, Education, and Law,* Volume XIX, Ablex Publishing, New Jersey.
Florida, R., (1994) "Buddhism and the Four Principles", in *Principles of Health Care Ethics,* Gillon, R., (ed.), John Wiley and Sons, Chichester.
Fontana, D., (1990) "Self-Assertion and Self-Transcendence in Buddhist Psychology", in *Space in Mind,* Crook, J. and Fontana, D., (eds.), Element Books, London.
Forbes, E., (1994) "Spirituality, Aging, and the Community-Dwelling Caregiver and Care Recipient", *Geriatric Nursing,* 15,6:297-302.
Forbis, P., (1988) "Meeting Patients' Spiritual Needs", *Geriatric Nursing,* May/June:158-159.
Fonow, M. and Cook, J., (eds.), (1991) *Beyond Methodology, Feminist Scholarship as Lived Research,* Indiana University Press, Bloomington.
Fonow, M. and Cook, J., (1991) "Back to the Future: A Look at the Second Wave of Feminist Epistemology and Methodology", in *Beyond Methodology,* Fonow, M. and Cook., Indiana University Press, Bloomington.
Foss, L., (1989) "The Challenge to Biomedicine: A Foundations Perspective",

Journal of Medicine and Philosophy, 14:165-191.
Foster, H., (1985) *Recodings: Art, Spectacle, Cultural Politics,* Bay Press, Washington.
Foucault, M., (1972) *The Archeology of Knowledge,* Routledge, London.
Foucault, M., (1973) *The Birth of the Clinic,* Vintage Books, New York.
Foucault, M., (1980) *Power/Knowledge,* Pantheon, New York.
Foucault, M., (1986) "What is Enlightenment?", *The Foucault Reader,* Rabinow, P., (ed.), Penguin, Harmondsworth.
Fox, M., (1990) *A Spirituality Named Compassion and the Healing of the Global Village, Humpty Dumpty and Us,* Harper, San Fancisco.
Fox, N., (1991) "Postmodernism, Rationality and the Evaluation of Health Care", *Sociological Review,* 39:709-744.
Fox, N., (1993) *Postmodernism, Sociology and Health,* Open University Press, Buckingham.
Fox, R., (1994) "How Did Bioethics Come To Be As It Is? An American Perspective", *Australian Bioethics Association, Third National Conference,* Unpublished Paper, Adelaide.
Frankl, V., (1973) *The Doctor and the Soul,* Vintage Books, New York.
Fraser, N. and Nicholson, L., (1988) "Social Criticism Without Philosophy: An Encounter Between feminism and Postmodernism", *Theory, Culture and Society,* 5,2-3:373-394.
Freidson, E., (1970) *Profession of Medicine, A Study of the Sociology of Applied Knowledge,* Dodd, Mead and Company, New York.
Freund, P. and McGuire, M., (1991) *Health, Illness, and the Social Body: A Critical Sociology,* Prentice Hall, Englewood Cliffs, N.J.
Fritschi, L. and Taylor, R., (1995) "Cancer - The Major Cause of Premature Mortality in Australia", *Cancer Forum,* 19,2:151-155.
Fromm, E., Suzuki, D. and De Martino, R., (1960) *Zen Buddhism and Psychoanalysis,* Souvenir Press, London.
Fuchs, V., (1968) "The Growing Demand for Medical Care", *New England Journal of Medicine,* 279,4:190-195.
Fullbrook, P., (1992) "Assessing Quality of Life: the Basis for Withdrawal of Life-Supporting Treatment?", *Journal of Advanced Nursing,* 17:1440-1446.
Fulton, R., (1972) "Death and Dying: Some Sociologic Aspects of Terminal care", *Modern Medicine,* May,29:74-77.
Fulton, R. and Owen, G., (1981) "Hospice in America", in *Hospice: The Living Idea,* Saunders, C., Summers, D. and Teller, N., (eds.), Edward Arnold, London.
Galloway, R., (1992) "A Teenager's Experience", *Oncology Nurse's Conference,* Unpublished Paper, Brisbane.
Gare, A., (1995) *Postmodernism and the Environmental Crisis,* Routledge, London.
Gatens, M., (1986) "Feminism, Philosophy and Reddles Without Answers", in *Feminist Challenges,* Pateman, C. and Gross, E., (eds.), Allen and Unwin, Sydney.
Gerteis, M., (ed.), (1993) *Through the Patient's Eyes, Understanding and Promoting Patient-Centered Care,* Jossey-Bass Publishers, San Francisco.

Gibson, M., (1976) "Rationality", *Philosophy and Public Affairs,* 6,3:193-225.
Gillett, G., (1989) "Informed Consent and Moral Integrity", *Journal of Medical Ethics,* 15:117-123.
Gillis, J., Tibballs, J., McEniery, J., Heavens, J., Hutchins, P., Kilham, H. and Henning, R., (1989) "Ventilator-Dependent Children", *The Medical Journal of Australia,* 150,2/2:10-14.
Gillon, R., (1988) "Living Wills, Posers of Attorney and Medical Practice", *Journal of Medical Ethics,* 14:59-60.
Gillon, R., (ed.), (1994) *Principles of Health Care Ethics,* John Wiley and Sons, Chichester.
Glaser, B. and Strauss, A., (1965) *Awareness of Dying,* Aldine, Chicago.
Gochman, D. and Bonham, G., (1988) "Physicians and the Hospice Decision: Awareness, Discussion, Reasons and Satisfaction", *The Hospice Journal,* 4,1:25-53.
Gochman, D. and Bonham, G., (1990) "The Social Structure of the Hospice Decision", *The Hospice Journal,* 6,1:15-36.
Goffman, E., (1968) *Asylums,* Penguin, Harmondsworth, Middlesex.
Goodin, E., (1988) "Heroic Measures and False Hopes", in *Philosophy and Medical Welfare,* Bell, J. and Mendus, S., (eds.), Cambridge University Press, Cambridge.
Goodloe, N. and Arreola, P., (1992) "Spiritual Health: Out of the Closet", *Journal of Health and Education,* May/June, 23,4:221-226.
Goodman, N., (1991) "Resource Allocation: Idealism, Realism, Pragmatism, Openness", *Journal of Medical Ethics,* 17:179-180.
Gotay, C., (1983) "Models of Terminal Care: A Review of the Research Literature", *Clinical and Investigative Medicine,* 6:131-41.
Greaves, D., (1989) "The Future Prospects for Living Wills", *Journal of Medical Ethics,* 15:179-182.
Green, J., Murton, F. and Statham, H., (1993) "Psychosocial Issues Raised By a Familial Ovarian Cancer Register", *Journal of Medical Genetics,* 30:575-579.
Green, R., (1990) "Method in Bioethics: A Troubled Assessment", *The Journal of Medicine and Philosophy,* 15:179-197.
Greer, D., (1985) "Hospice: From Social Movement to Health Care Industry", *Transactions of the American Clinical and Climatological Association,* 97:82-87.
Greer, D., Mor, V., Morris, J., Sherwood, S., Kidder, D. and Birnbaum, H., (1986) "An Alternative in Terminal Care: Results of the National Hospice Study", *Journal of Chronic Diseases,* 39,1:9-26.
Griffin, A., (1993) "Holism in Nursing: Its Meaning and Value", *British Journal of Nursing,* 2,6:310-312.
Grof, S. and Grof, C., (eds.), (1989) *Spiritual Emergency, When Personal Transformation Becomes a Crises,* Jeremy P. Tarcher, Los Angeles.
Gunew, S., (1990) *Feminist Knowledge : Critique and Construct,* Routledge, New York.
Guralnik, D., (ed.), (1982) *Webster's New World Dictionary,* 2nd Edition, Simon and Schuster, New York.

Haines, K., Zalcberg J. and Buchanan, J., (1990) "Not-for Resuscitation Orders in Cancer Patients - Principles of Decision-Making", *The Medical Journal of Australia,* 153,20/8:225-229.

Hamilton, M. and Reid, H., (1980) *A Hospice Handbook: A New Way to Care for the Dying,* William B Eerdmans Publishing Company, Grand Rapids.

Ham-Ying, S., (1993) "Analysis of the Concept of Holism Within the Context of Nursing", *British Journal of Nursing,* 2,15:771-775.

Harding, S., (1986) *The Science Question in Feminism,* Cornell Paperbacks, London.

Harding, S., (ed.), (1987) *Feminism and Methodology,* Indiana University Press, Indianopolis.

Harding, S., (1987) "Introduction: Is There a Feminist Method?" in *Feminism and Methodology,* (ed.), Harding, S., Indiana University Press, Indianapolis.

Harding, S., (1990) "Feminsim, Science, and the Anti-Enlightenment Critiques", in *Feminism, Postmodernism,* Nicholson, L., (ed.), Routledge, New York.

Hart, N., (1985) *The Sociology of Health and Medicine,* Causeway Books, Lancashire.

Hawking, S., (1988) *A Brief History of Time,* Bantam, London.

Hecht, A. and Moser, D., (1991) "Organisational Evolution: A Hospice Case Study", *The Hospice Journal,* 7,3:57-71.

Heisenberg, W., (1962) *Physics and Philsophy,* Harper and Row, New York.

Hewa, S. and Hetherington, R., (1990) "Specialists Without Spirit:Crisis in the Nursing Profession", *Journal of Medical Ethics,* 16:179-184.

Highfield, M., (1992) "Spiritual Health of Oncology Patients: Nurse and patient Perspectives", *Cancer Nursing,* 15,1:1-8.

Highfield, M. and Carson, C., (1983) "Spiritual Needs of Patients: Are They Recognised", *Cancer Nursing,* 6,3:187-192.

Holman, E., (1990) "Death and the Health Professional: Organisation and Defense in Health Care", *Death Studies,* 14:13-24.

Holmes, H. and Purdy, L., (1992) *Feminist Perspectives in Medical Ethics,* Indiana University Press, Indianapolis.

Holmes, R., (1990) "The Limited Relevance of Analytical Ethics to the Problems of Bioethics", *The Journal of Medicine and Philosophy,* 15:143-159.

Horkheimer, M., (1978) "The End of Reason", in *The Essential Frankfurt School Reader,* Arato, A. and Gebhardt, E., (eds.), Urizen Books, New York.

Howe, A., (1982) "Beginning at the End: Patterns of Death Among the Aged", *Community Health Studies,*6,3,:253-262.

Hull, M., (1991) "Hospice Nurses: Caring Support for Caregiving Families", *Cancer Nursing,* 14,2:63-70.

Humphreys, C., (1977) *The Buddhist Way of Action: A Working Philosophy for Daily Life,* George Allen and Unwin, London.

Hunt, M., (1992) "Scripts' for dying at home - displayed in nurses', patients' and relatives' talk", *Journal of Advanced Nursing,* 17,1297-1302.

Huyssen, A., (1987) "Foreward: The Return of Diogenes as Postmodern

Intellectual", in *Critique of Cynical Reason,* Sloterdijk, P., (Trans. Eldred, M.,), University of Minnesota Press, Minneapolis.
Huyssen, A., (1990) "Mapping the Postmodern", in *Feminism, Postmodernism,* Nicholson, L., (ed.), Routledge, New York.
Hyman, R. and Bulkin, W., (1990) "Physician Reported Incentives and Disincentives for Referring patients to Hospice", *The Hospice Journal,* 6,4:39-59.
Illich, I., (1976) *Medical Nemesis,* Pantheon Books, New York.
Isaacs, P., (1993) "What is Philosophy?" *Lecture Summary, HUB003,* Queensland University of Technology, Brisbane.
Jackson, D. and Soothill, R., (1989) *Is The Medicine Making You Ill,* Angus and Robertson, North Rhyde.
Jacob, J., (1988) *Doctors and Rules,* Routledge, London.
Jaggar, A., (1991) "Feminist Ethics: Projects, Prolems, Prospects", in *Feminist Ethics,* Card, C., (ed.), University of Kansas, Kansas.
James, N. and Field, D., (1986) "The Routinization of Hospice: Charisma and Bureaucratization", *Social Science and Medicine,* 34,12:1363-1375.
Jameson, F., (1984) *Postmodernism, or the Cultural Logic of Late Capitalism,* Duke University Press, Durham.
Jecker, N., (1991a) "Knowing When to Stop: The Limits of Medicine", *Hastings Center Report,* May-June:5-8.
Jecker, N., (1991b) "Separating Care and Cure: An Analysis of Historical and Contemporary Images of Nursing and Medicine", *The Journal of Medicine and Philosophy,* 16:285-306.
Jecker, N. and Schneiderman, L., (1995) "When Families Request that 'Everything Possible' Be Done", *The Journal of Medicine and Philosophy,*20:145-163.
Jeffrey, D., (1993) *'There is Nothing More I Can Do':An Introduction to the Ethics of Palliative Care,* The Pattern Press, Cornwell.
Jennett, B., (1986) *High Technology Medicine, Benefits and Burdens,* Oxford University Press, Oxford.
Jennett, B., (1992) "Health Technology Assessment", *British Medical Journal,* 305:67-68.
Jennett, B., (1994) "Medical Technology, Social and Health Care Issues", in *Principles of Health Care Ethics,* Gillon, R., (ed), John Wiley and Sons, Chichester.
Jensen, U. and Mooney, G., (eds.), (1990) *Changing Values in Medical and Health Care Decision Making,* John Wiley and Sons, West Sussex.
Johnson, A., (1990) *Pathways in Medical Ethics,* Edward Arnold, London.
Johnstone, M., (1994) *Bioethics : A Nursing Perspective,* 2nd Ed., Harcourt Brace Jovanovich, Marrickville.
Jones, B., (1988) "Psychological Adjustment After Cardiac Transplantation", *The Medical Journal of Australia,* 149,1/8:118-122.
Jones, D., (1989) "The New Zealand Report of the Cervical Cancer Inquiry: Significance For Medical Education", *The Medical Journal of Australia,* 151,16/10:454-456.
Jonsen, A., (1990) *The New Medicine and the Old Ethics,* Harvard University

Press, London.
Joseph, K., (1993) "Health Care Resources: A History of the Debate", *Bioethics Outlook,* 4,4:1-4,8.
Jung, C., (1955) *Modern Man in Search of Soul,* Harcourt Brace Jovanovich, London.
Kaczorowski, J., (1989) "Spiritual Well-Being and Anxiety in Adults Diagnosed with Cancer", *The Hospice Journal,* 5,3/4:105-116.
Kalupahana, D., (1976) *Buddhist Philosophy, A Historical Analysis,* University of Hawaii Press, Honolulu.
Kane, R., (1986) "Lessons From Hospice Evaluations", *Hospice Journal,* 2,3:3-8.
Kant, I., (1964) *The Doctrine of Virtue: Part 11 of the Metaphysics of Morals,* (trans. Gregory, M.), New York.
Kass, L., (1991) "Death with Dignity and the Sanctity of Life" in *The Ethics of Choice: A time to be Born and a Time to Die,* (ed.), Kogan, B., Aldine De Gruyter, New York.
Kaye, R. and Robinson, K., (1994) "Caregivers", *Image, Journal of Nursing Scholarship,* 26,3:218-221.
Kearsley, J., Hirst, C., (1991) "Breast Cancer Screening : 'One Swallow Doth Not a Summer Make'", *The Medical Journal of Australia,* 154,21/1:76-78.
Kearsley, J., (1993) "Spiritual Pain - The Pain Only The Self Can Heal", *Spiritual Pain in Health Care Seminar,* Unpublished paper, Karuna Hospice Service, Brisbane.
Kellehear, A., (1990) *Dying of Cancer, The Final Year of Life,* Harwood Academic Publishers, London.
Kellner, K., (1988) "Postmodernism as Social Theory: Some Challenges and Problems", *Theory, Culture and Society,* 5,2-3:239-270.
Kennedy, I., (1981) *The Unmasking of Medicine,* Allen and Unwin, London.
Kessler, D., (1991) "Drug Promotion and Scientific Exchange: The Role of the Clinical Investigation", *The New England Journal of Medicine,* 325,3:201-203.
Kieffer, G., (1979) *Bioethics: A Textbok of Issues,* Addison-Wells, Philippines.
King, K., (1987) "Health Law and Ethics", *The Medical Journal of Australia,* 146,5/1:22-26.
King, M., Speck, P. and Thomas, A., (1994) "Spiritual and Religious Beliefs in Acute Illness-Is This a Feasible Area For Study?", *Social Science and Medicine,* 38,4:631-636.
Kirschling, J. and Pittman, J., (1989) "Measurement of Spiritual Well-being: A Hospice Caregiver Sample", *The Hospice Journal,* 5,2:1-11.
Klagsbrun, S., (1981) "Hospice - A Developing Role", in *Hospice: The Living Idea,* Saunders, C., Summers, D. and Teller, N., (eds.), Edward Arnold, London.
Klein, R., (1992) "The Unethics of Hormone Replacement Therapy", *Bioethics News,* 11,3:24-37.
Kleinman, S., (1986) *Mind and Body: East meets West,* Human Kinetics Publishers, Illinois.
Kliever, L., (ed.), (1989) *Dax's Case, Essays in Medical Ethics and Human*

Meaning, Southern Methodist University Press, Texas.
Koff, T., (1980) *Hospice: A Caring Community,* Winthrop Publishers, Cambridge, Massachusetts.
Kogan, B., (1991) *The Ethics of Choice: A Time to Be Born and a Time to Die,* Aldine De Gruyter, New York.
Kohut, J. and Kohut, S., (1984) *Hospice: Caring for the Terminally Ill,* Charles C Thomas Publisher, Springfield, Illinois.
Komesaroff, P., (1996) *Troubled Bodies: Critical Perspectives on Postmodernism, Medical Ethics and the Body,* Melbourne University Press, Melbourne.
Koestler, A., (1967) *The Ghost in the Machine,* Arkana, London.
Krant, M., (1974) *Dying and Dignity: The Meaning and Control of a Personal Death,* Charles C Thomas Publisher, Springfield, Illinois, USA.
Kubler-Ross, E., (1969) *On Death and Dying,* Macmillan,New York.
Kubler-Ross, E., (1974) *Questions and Answers on Death and Dying,*Macmillan Publishing, New York.
Kubler-Ross, E., (1975) *Death: The Final Stage of Growth,* Prentice Hall, Englewood Cliffs, NJ.
Kutscher, A., Klagsbrun, S., Torpie, R., DeBellis, R., Hale, M. and Tallmer, M., (eds.), (1983) *Hospice USA,* Columbia University Press, New York.
Labun, E., (1988) "Spiritual Care: An Element in Nursing Care Planning",*Journal of Advanced Nursing,* 13:314-320.
Lafer, B., (1991) "The Attrition of Hospice Volunteers", *Omega,* 23,3:161-168.
Lamers, W., (1988) "Hospice Research: Some Reflections", *The Hospice Journal,* 4,3:3-11.
La Monica., Madea, A. & Oberst, M., (1987) "Empathy and Nursing Care Outcomes", *Scholarly Inquiry for Nursing Practice: An International Journal,* 1,3:197-213.
Lather, P., (1986) "Research as Praxis", *Harvard Educational Review,* 56,3:257-277.
Lather, P., (1986) "Issues of Validity in Openly Ideological Research: Between a Rock and a Soft Place", *Interchange,* 17,4:63-84.
Lather, P., (1989) "Deconstructing/deconstructive Inquiry: Issues in Feminist Research Methodologies", Paper Presented at the New Zealand Women's Studies Association Conference, Christchurch.
Lather, P., (1991) *Getting Smart: Feminist Research and Pedogogy With/in the Postmodern,* Routledge, New York.
Lather, P., (1992) "Critical Frames in Educational Research: Feminist and Post-structural Perspectives", *Theory and Practice,* xxxi,2:87-97.
Lazarus, R. and Leeder, S., (1989) "Technology in Health Care - You Don't Need a Lithotriptor to Solve the Problem of Cracking Nuts", *The Medical Journal of Australia,*151,17/7:38-40.
Lebacqz, K., (1992) "Humility in Health Care", *The Journal of Medicine and Philosophy,*17:291-307.
Leeder, S., (1989) "The Ethics of Rationing Health-Care Resources", *The Medical Journal of Australia,* 151,6/11.

Lemert, C., (1992) "General Social Theory, Irony, Postmodernism", in *Postmodernism & Social Theory,* Seidman, S. and Wagner, D., (eds.), Basil Blackwell, Cambridge.
Lerman, C., Trock, ., Rimer, B., Boyce, A., Jepson, C. and Engstrom, P., (1991) "Psychological and Behavioral Implications of Abnormal Mammograms", *Annals of Internal Medicine,* 114,8:657-661.
Levy, J., (1982) "The Staging of Negotiations Between Hospice and Medical Institutions", *Urban Life,* 11,3:293-311.
Lockwood, M., (ed.), (1985a) *Moral Dilemmas in Modern Medicine,* Oxford University Press, Oxford.
Lockwood, M., (1985b) "The Warnock Report: A Philosophical Appraisal", in *Moral Dilemmas in Modern Medicine,* Oxford University Press, Oxford.
Lorber, J., (1989) "Choice, Gift, or Patriarchal Bargain? Women's Consent to In Vitro Fertilization in Male Infertility", *Hypatia,* 4,3:23-36.
Lowe, I., (1989) "Choosing Health Care Technologies", *New Doctor,* 51:10-14.
Lumby, J., (1994) *Exploring the Experience of a Life-Threatening Illness,* New England Press, Armidale.
Lustig, A., (1992) "The Method of 'Principlism': A Critique of the Critique", *The Journal of Medicine and Philosophy,* 17:487-510.
Lyotard, J-F., (1984) *The Postmodern Condition: A Report on Knowledge,* Manchester University Press, Manchester.
MacCormack, C., (1994) "Editorial: Hospice and the Holistic Alternative", *Social Science and Medicine,* 38,11:vii-ix.
MacDonald, D., (1989) "Non-admissions: The Other Side of the Hospice Story", *The American Journal of Hospice Care,* 6,2:17-19.
MacDonald, D., (1990) "Hospice, Entropy, and the 1990's: Toward a Hospice World View", *The American Journal of Hospice and Palliative Care,* 7:39-47.
MacDonald, I., (1989) "New Technology For Old?", *The Medical Journal of Australia,* 151,3/7:3-5.
MacIntyre, A., (1985) *After Virtue: A Study in Moral Theory,* Duckworth, London.
Malden, L., Sutherland, C., Tattersall, M., Moragan, J., Forsyth, S., Levi, J., Gunz, F., (1984) "Dying of Cancer: Factors Influencing the Place of Death of Patients", *Medical Journal of Australia,* 141,3:147-150.
Mandel, T., (1993) "Future Directions in Transplantation", *The Medical Journal of Australia,* 158:269-272.
Manning, M., (1984) *The Hospice Alternative: Living with Dying,* Souvenir Press, London.
Mappes, T. and Zembaty, J., (1991) *Biomedical Ethics,* McGraw-Hill, New York.
Marcuse, H., (1972) *One Dimensional Man,* Abacus, London.
Martocchio, B., (1982) *Living While Dying,* Prentice-Hall, Maryland.
Maseide, P., (1991) "Possibly Abusive, Often Benign, and Always Necessary. On Power and Domination in Medical Practice", *Sociology of Health and Illness,* 13,4:545-561.

May, W., (1991) *The Patient's Ordeal,* Indiana University Press, Bloomington.
May, W., (1994) "On the Many Voices of Bioethics", *Hastings Center Report,* May-June:26-27
McCarl Nielsen, J., (ed.), (1990) *Feminist Research Methods,* Westview Press, Sydney.
McCracken, G., (1988) *The Long Interview,* Qualitative Research Methods Series 13, A Sage University Paper, London.
McGrath, P., (1992) "Chemotherapy : The Ethic of an Illusion", *Second National Bioethics Conference,* Proceedings, Plennary Session, Sydney.
McGrath, P., (1993) "The Implications of the 'Semiotics of Hope' in Relation to Chemotherapy", *New Doctor,* Summer:21-25.
McGrath, P., (1994) "It's OK to Say No!: A Discussion of Ethical Issues Arising From Informed Consent to Chemotherapy", *Cancer Nursing,* 18,1/2.
McGrath, P., (1994) "If Only It Had Been - 'Sentio Ego Sum'!: The Role of Emotion in Ethical Reasoning", *Third National Bioethics Conference, Proceedings,* Adelaide.
McGrath, P. and Turner, G., (1995) "The Ethics of Hope: Newspaper Reporting of Chemotherapy", *Australian Studies in Journalism,* 4:50-71.
McGrath, P. and Kearsley, J., (1995) "Is There a Better Way? Bioethical Reflections on Palliative Cytotoxic Drug Use", *Palliative Medicine,* 9:269-271.
McGrath, P., (1996) "The Question of Choice: A Bioethical Perspective on Chemotherapy", *Cancer Forum,* 20,2:113-116.
McGrath, P. & Markman, M., (1996) "Bioethical Reflections on the Limitations of Cytotoxic Drug Use", *Monash Bioethics Review,* 15,4:9-14.
McInerney, F., (1992) "Provision of Food and Fluids in Terminal Care: a Sociological Analysis", *Social Science and Medicine,* 34,11:1271-1276.
McNulty, E. and Holderby, R., (1983) *Hospice: A Caring Challenge,* Charles C Thomas Publishers, Springfield, USA.
Mehlman, M., (1986) "Health Care Cost Containment and Medical Technology: A Critique of Waste Theory", *Case Western Reserve Law Review,* 36:778-877.
Melski, J., (1992) "Price of Technology", *Journal of American Medical Association,* 267,11,18/3:1516-1518.
Menzel, P., (1990) *Strong Medicine: The Ethical Rationing of Health Care,* Oxford University Press, New York.
Miller, R. and Rahr, H., (1983) *Social Work Issues in Health Care,* Prentice-Hall, Englewood Cliffs, N.J.
Millison, M. and Dudley, J., (1990) "The Importance of Spirituality in Hospice Work: A Study of Hospice Professionals", *The Hospice Journal,* 6,3:63-77.
Millison, M. and Dudley, J., (1992) "Providing Spiritual Support: A Job for All Hospice Professionals", *The Hospice Journal,* 8,4:49-66.
Mishler, E., (1981) "Viewpoint: Critical Perspectives on the Biomedical Model", *Social Contexts of Health, Illness and Patient Care,* Mishler, E., Amarasingham, L., Osherson, S., Hauser, S., Waxler, N., Liem, R., (eds)., Cambridge University Press, Cambridge.
Mishler, E., (1984) *The Discourse of Medicine. Dialectics of Medical*

Interviews, Ablex, Norwood, N.J.
Mitchell, K. and Lovat, T., (1991) *Bioethics for Medical and Health Professionals,* Social Science Press, Wentworth Falls.
Miyaja, N., (1993) "The Power of Compassion: Truth-Telling Among American Doctors in the Care of Dying Patients", *Social Science and Medicine,* 36,3:249-264.
Montgomery, M., (1995) "One and a Half Hours a Week...", *The Karuna Hospice News,* 1-2.
Mor, B., Greer, D. and Kastenbaum, R., (1988) *The Hospice Experiment,.* The Johns Hopkins University Press, Baltimore.
Moran, R., (1991) "Working with Doctors, Different Priorities", *Nursing Times,* June 26, 87,26:35-37.
Morgan, K., (1988) "Women and Moral Madness", in *Feminist Perspectives: Philosophical Essays on Methods and Morals,* Code, L., Mullett, S. and Overall, C., (eds.), University of Toronto Press, Toronto.
Morison, R., (1975a) "Death: Process or Event?", in *Hastings Center Report, Death Inside Out,* Harper and Row, New York.
Morison, R., (1975b) "The Dignity of the Inevitable and Necessary", in *Hastings Center Report, Death Inside Out,* Harper and Row, New York.
Morreim, J., (1985) "Cost Containments Issues of Moral Conflict and Justice for Physicians", *Theoretical Medicine,* 6,6:257-279.
Morreim, E., (1987) "Cost Containments and the Standard Medical Care", *California Law Review,* 75:1719-63.
Morse, G., Anderson, G., Bottorff, J., Yonge, O., O"Brien, S., Solberg, S. & McIlveen, K., (1992) "Exploring Empathy: A Conceptual Model for Nursing Care", *IMAGE: Journal of Nursing Scholarship,* 24,4:273-280.
Moulton, J., (1983) "A Paradigm of Philosophy: The Adversary Method" in *Discovering Reality,* Harding, S. and Hintrikka, M., (eds.), D. Reidel, Dordrecht.
Mount, B., (1985) "Challenges in Palliative Care", *The American Journal of Hospice Care,* 2,6:22-29.
Mulkay, M., (1985) *The Word and the World: explorations in the Form of Sociological Analysis,* George Allen and Unwin, London.
Mumby, D., (1988) *Communication and Power in Organizations: Discourse, Ideology, and Domination,* Ablex Publishing Corporation, New Jersey.
Mumby, D. and Stohl, C., (1991) "Power and Discourse in Organization Studies: Absence and the Dialetic of Control", *Discourse & Society,* 2,3:313-332.
Munley, A., (1983) *The Hospice Alternative: A New Context for Death and Dying,* Basic Books, New York.
Nagai-Jacobson, M. and Burkhardt, M., (1989) "Spirituality:cornerstone of Holistic Nursing Practice", *Holistic Nursing Practice,* 3,3:18-26.
Navarro, V., (1976) *Medicine Under Capitalism,* Prodist, New York.
Navarro, V., (1986) *Crisis, Health and Medicine, A Social Critique,* Tavistock Publications, London.
Nelson, R. and Drought, T., (1992) "Justice and the Moral Acceptability of Rationing Medical Care: The Oregon Experiment", *Journal of Medicine and*

Philosophy, 17:97-117.
Newell, C., (1991) "A Critical Evaluation of the NH & MRC's "The Ethics of Limiting Life-sustaining Treatment" and Related Perspectives on Disability and Bioethics", *Bioethics and a Wider Community*, First Annual Conference of the Australian Bioethics Association, University of Melbourne.
Newell, C., (1992) "The Ethics of the Cochlear Implant: Conflict and the Role of Culture in Formulating Knowledge and Ethical Discourse", *Australian Bioethics Association Second Annual Conference*, Proceedings, Sydney University, Sydney, Plenary Session, Volume 1.
Newell, C., (1994) "Towards an Ethics of Resources Allocation for Australian Disability Services", *Bioethics 1971-2001*, Proceedings of Australian Bioethics Association Third Annual Conference, Adelaide University Union, Adelaide.
Newell, C., (1994) "A Critique of the Construction of Prenatal Diagnosis and Disability", in *The Proceedings of the Conference: Ethical Issues in Prenatal Diagnosis and the Termination of Pregnancy*, McKie, J., (ed.), Centre for Human Bioethics, Monash University, Melbourne:89-96.
Newell, C., (1995) "Ethics in and of Communities: The Ethical Worlds and Discourses of General Practitioners and Consumers with Disabilities", *Autonomy, Community and Justice in Bioethics*, Proceedings Fourth National Australian Bioethics Association Conference, St John"s College, University of Queensland, Brisbane.
Nicholson, R., (1994) "Limitations of the Four Principles", in *Principles of Health Care Ethics*, Gillon, R., (ed.), John Wiley and Sons, Chichester.
Nicolson, M. and McLaughlin, C., (1987) "Social Constructionism and Medical Sociology: A Reply to M. R. Bury", *Sociology of Health and Illness*, 9,2:107-126.
Noddings, N., (1984) *Caring; A Feminine Approach to Ethics and Moral Education*, University of California Press, Berkeley.
Norris, C., (1982) *Deconstruction: Theory and Practice*, Methuen, London.
Norris, C., (1987) *Derrida*, Fontana Press, London.
Norris, C., (1989) *Deconstruction and the Interests of Theory*, University of Oklahoma Press, London.
Nuland, S., (1994) *How We Die: Reflections on Life"s Final Chapter*, Alfred A. Knopf, New York.
Oldroyd, D., (1986) *The Arch of Knowledge*, New South Wales University Press, Kensington.
Otlowski, M., (1995) "Legal and Ethical Issues in Palliative Care", *Monash Bioethics Review*, 4,1:33-47.
Page, M., (1989) *The Tao of Power: An Eastern Way to a Greener World*, Green Print, London.
Paige, G. and Gilliatt, S., (eds.), (1991) *Buddhism and Nonviolent Global Problem-Solving*, Center for Global Nonviolence Planning Project Spark M. Matsunaga Institute for Peace, University of Hawaii, Honolulu.
Palmer, G. and Short, S., (1989) *Health Care and Public Policy*, The Macmillan Company of Australia, Crows Nest.
Paradis, L. and Cummings, S., (1986) "The Evolution of Hospice in America

Toward Organizational Homogeneity", *Journal of Health and Social Behaviour*,27,370-386.
Paradis, L., (ed.), (1987) *Stress and Burnout Among Providers Caring for the Terminally Ill and Their Families,* The Haworth Press, London.
Paradis, L., (1988) "An Assessment of Sociology's Contributions to Hospice: Priorities for Future Research", *The Hospice Journal,* 4,3:57-71.
Parise, I. and Meers, G., (1986) "Low Morale in Public Hospitals", *New Doctor,* 39:18-20.
Parsons, T., (1951) *The Social System,* Routledge and Kegan Paul, London.
Patchner, M. and Finn, M., (1987) "Volunteers: The Life-Line of Hospice", *Omega,* 18,2:135-144.
Pattison, E., (1977) *The Experience of Dying,* Prentice-Hall, Englewood Cliffs, N.J.
Patton, P., (1986) "Ethics and Postmodernity" in *Futer Fall: Excursions into Postmodernity,* Grosz, E., Threadgold, T., Kelly, D., Cholodenko, A. and Colless, E., (eds.), Power Institute Sydney University, Sydney.
Pawley, M., (1986) "Architecture: All the History That Fits", *Guardian,* 3/12:10.
Pearson, A., (1993a) "Nursing, Technology and the Human Condition", *Journal of Advanced Nursing,* Guest Editorial, 18:165-167.
Pearson, I., (1993b) "The Potential Organ Donor", *The Medical Journal of Australia,* 158:45-47.
Peile, C., (1994) "Theory, Practice, Research: Casual Acquaintances or a Seamless Whole?" *Australian Social Work,* 47,2:17-23.
Pellegrino, E., (1979) *Humanism and the Physician,* The University of Tennessee Press, Knoxville.
Pellegrino, E. and Thomasma, D., (1988) *For the Patient's Good: The Restoration of Beneficence in Health Care,* Oxford University Press, Oxford.
Pelletier, K., (1990) *Holistic Medicine: From Stress to Optimum Health,* Peter Smith, Gloucester, Mass.
Perakyla, A., (1989) "Appealing to the "Experience" of the Patient in the Care of the Dying", *Sociology of Health and Illness,* 11,2:117-134.
Petersen, A., (1994) *In a Critical Condition, Health and Power Relations in Australia,* Allen and Unwin, St Leonards, NSW.
Petrosino, B., (ed.), (1986) *Nursing in Hospice and Palliative Care,* The Haworth Press, London.
Petrosino, B., (1988) "Nursing Research in Hospice Care", *The Hospice Journal,* 4,3:29-45.
Phillips, D., (1971) *Knowledge From What?: Theories and Methods in Social Research,* Rand McNally and Company, Chicago.
Pierce, C., (1991) "Postmodernism and Other Skepticism", in *Feminist Ethics,* Card, C., (ed.), University of Kansas, Kansas.
Plowles, J., (1973) "On the Limitations of Modern Medicine", *Social Science and Medicine,* 1:1-30.
Pollard, B., (1991) "Withdrawing Life-Sustaining Treatment from Severely Branin-Damaged Persons", *The Medical Journal of Australia,* 154,4/12:559-

561.
Pollock-Byrne, J., (1989) *Ethics in Crime and Justice: Dilemmas and Decisions,* Wadsworth, Belmont.
Poss,S., (1981) *Towards Death with Dignity,* George Allen and Unwin, London.
Pratt, D. and Filicky-Peneski, R., (1983) "Relating to the Dying: A Philosophy of Continuing Care", in *Hospice USA,* Kutscher, A., Kagsbrun, S., Torpic, R., De Bellis, R., Hale, M. and Tallmer, M., (eds.), Columbia University Press, New York.
Preston, T., (1981) *The Clay Pedestal,* Madrona Publishers, Seattle.
Punch, M., (1974) "The Sociology of the Anti-institution", *British Journal Sociology,* 25:312-325.
Rabinow, P., (ed.), (1984) *The Foucault Reader,* Penguin Books, Middlesex, England.
Raffin, T., Shurkin, J. and Sinkler, W., (1989) *Intensive Care: Facing the Critical Choices,* WH Freeman, New York.
Ramsey, P., (1975) "The Indignity of "Death With Dignity"", in *Hastings Center Report, Death Inside Out,* Harper and Row, New York.
Raphael, D., (1981) *Moral Philosophy,* Oxford University Press, Oxford.
Ratanakul, P., (1986) *Bio Ethics: An Introduction to the Ethics of Medicine and Life Sciences,* Mahidol University, Bangkok, Thailand.
Ratanakul, P., (1988) "Bioethics in Thailand: The Struggle for Buddhist Solutions", *The Journal of Medicine and Philosophy,* 13:301-312.
Ratcliff, K., Feree, M., Mellow, G., Wright, B., Price, G., Yanoshik, K. and Fenton, M., (ed.), (1989) *Healing Technology: Feminist Perspectives,* The University of Michigan Press, USA.
Ratcliff, K., (1989) "Health Technologies for Women: Whose Health? Whose Technology?", in *Health Technology,* Ratcliff, K., Feree, M., Mellow, G., Wright, B., Price, G., Yanoshik, K. and Fenton, M., (ed.), The University of Michigan Press, USA.
Raudonis, B., (1991), *A Nursing Study of Empathy from the Hospice Patient's Perspective,* Unpublished Doctoral Dissertation, University of Texas, Austin.
Raudonis, B., (1992) "Ethical Considerations in Qualitative Research with Hospice Patients", *The Hospice Journal,* 2,2:238-249.
Raudonis, B., (1995) "Empathic Nurse-Patient Relationships in Hospice Nursing", *The Hospice Journal,* 10 (1):59-73.
Rawlinson, M., (1987) "Foucault's Strategy: Knowledge, Power, and the Specificity of Truth", *The Journal of Medicine and Philosophy,* 12:371-395.
Relman, A., (1980) "The New Medical-Industrial Complex", *New England Journal of Medicine,* 303,17:963-970.
Restak, R., (1975) *Pre-Meditated Man: Bioethics and the Control of Future Human Life,* The Viking Press, New York.
Reynolds, F., (1978) "Death: Eastern Thought" in *Encyclopedia of Bioethics,* Reich, W., (ed.), Free Press, New York.
Rice, S., (1988) *Some Doctors Make You Sick,* Angus and Robertson, North Rhyde.
Rinaldi, A. and Kearl, M., (1990) "The Hospice Farewell: Ideological

Perspectives of Its Professional Practitioners", *Omega,* 21,4:283-300.
Rinpoche, S., (1992) *The Tibetan Book of Living and Dying,* Random House, Sydney.
Risjord, M., (1993) "Relativism and the Social Scientific Study of Medicine", *The Journal of Medicine and Philosophy,* 18:195-212.
Ritchie, K., (1988) "Professionalism, Altruism, and Overwork", *The Journal of Medicine and Philosophy,* 13:447-455.
Rorty, R., (1989) *Contingency, Irony, and Solidarity,* Cambridge University Press, Cambridge.
Ross, G., (1993) *The Search for the Pearl,* Australian Broadcasting Corporation, Sydney.
Ross, L., (1994) "Spiritual Aspects of Nursing", *Journal of Advanced Nursing,* 19:439-447.
Roth, J., (1979) "The Necessity and Control of Hospitalization", in *Health, Illness, and Medicine,* Albrecht, G. and Higgins, P., Rand McNally, Chicago.
Rowland, R., (1992) "An Ethical Response to Reproductive Technology", *Australian and New Zealand Association for the Advancement of Science Conference,* Unpublished paper, Brisbane.
Russell, B., (1946) *History of Western Philosophy,* Routledge, London.
Russell, G., (1989) "Hospice Programs and the Hospice Movement: An Investigation Based on General Systems Theory", *The Hospice Journal,* 5,3/4:23-49.
Rutten, F. and Bonsel, G., (1992) "High cost Technology in Health Care: A Benefit or a Burden?", *Social Science and Medicine,* 35,4:567-577.
Ryomin, A., (1990) *New Mahayana, Buddhism for a Post-Modern World,* Asian Humanities Press, Berkeley, California.
Sabatino, C., (1993) "Surely the Wizard Will Help Us, Toto? Implementing the Patient Self-Determination Act", *Hastings Center Report,* January/ February:12-16.
Saunders, C., (1981a) "The Founding Philosophy" in *Hospice: The Living Idea,* Saunders, C., Summers, D. and Teller, N., (eds.), Edward Arnold, London.
Saunders, C., (1981b) "The Hospice: Its Meaning to Patients and Their Physicians", *Hospital Practice,* June:93-108.
Saunders, C., (ed.), (1984) *The Management of Terminal Malignant Disease,* Edward Arnold, London.
Saunders, C., (1993) "Forward", in *Oxford Textbook of Palliative Medicine,* Doyle, D., Hanks, G. and Macdonald, N., (eds.), Oxford University Press, Oxford.
Saunders, C., (1994) "The Dying Patient", in *Principles of Health Care Ethics,* Gillon, R., (ed.), John Wiley and Sons, Chichester.
Saunders, C. and Baines, M., (1983) *Living with Dying: The Management of Terminal Disease,* Oxford University Press, Oxford.
Saunders, C., Summers, D. and Teller, N., (eds.), (1981) *Hospice: The Living Idea,* Edward Arnold, London.
Scarlett, B., (1994) "On the Death of Tony Bland", *Res Publica,* 3,2:14-17.
Scofield, G., (1991a) "Is Consent Useful When Resuscitation Isn"t?", *Hastings*

Center Report, November/December:28-35.
Scofield, G., (1991b) "Organ and Tissue Transplantation", *The Medical Journal of Australia, 154,20/5:643-644.*
Schel, B., (1989) "Ethics of Caring and the Institutional Ethics Committee", *Hypatia,* 4, 2:45-56.
Scott, C., (1987) "The Power of Medicine, The Power of Ethics", *Journal of Medicine and Philosophy,* 12:336-350.
Seffrin, J., Wilson, J. and Black, B., (1991) "Patient Perceptions" *Cancer,* March 15 Supplement, 67:1783-1787.
Siebers, T., (1988) *The Ethics of Criticism,* Cornell University Press, London.
Siebold, C., (1992) *The Hospice Movement: Easing Death's Pains,* Twayne Publishers, New York.
Seibold, D., Rossi, S., Berteotti, C., Soprych, S. and McQuillan, L., (1987) "Volunteer Involvement in a Hopsice Care Program", *American Journal of Hospice Care,* 4,3:44-55.
Seidman, S. and Wagner, D., (eds.), (1992) *Postmodernism & Social Theory,* Basil Blackwell, Cambridge.
Seidman, S., (1992) "Postmodern Social Theory as Narrative with a Moral Intent", in *Postmodernism & Social Theory,* Seidman, S. and Wagner, D., (eds.), Basil Blackwell, Cambridge.
Shaw, L., Miler, J., Slutsky, A., Maurer, J., Puskas, J., Patterson, A. and Singer, P., (1991) "Ethics of Lung Transplantation With Live Donors", *The Lancet,* 338:678-681.
Sherson, S., (1991) "Nursing Reflections on Transplantation", *Proceedings from the Australian Bioethics First Annual Conference, Bioethics and the Wider Community,* Melbourne.
Shenkin, H., (1991) *Medical Ethics: Evolution, Rights and the Physician,* Kluwer Academic Publishers, Dordrecht.
Short, S., (1985) "The War Against Cancer: A Sociological Study of Cancer Treatment", *New Doctor,* March, 35:25-28.
Shusterman, R., (1988) "Postmodernist Aestheticism: A New Moral Philosophy?" , *Theory, Culture and Society,*5,2-3:337-356.
Sims, C., (1987) "Spiritual Care As a Part of Holistic Nursing", *Imprint,* 34,6:63-65.
Singer, P., Siegler, M., Whittington, P., Lantos, J., Emond, J., Thistlethwaite, J. and Broelsch, C., (1989) "Ethics of Liver Transplantation with Living Donors", *The New England Journal of Medicine,* 312:620-622.
Singer, P., (1993) "The International Association of Bioethics", *The Medical Journal of Australia,* 158:298-299.
Singer, P., (1994) *Rethinking Life and Death,* The Text Publishing Company, Melbourne.
Smart, B., (1993) *Postmodernity,* Routledge, London.
Smith, E., Stefanek, M., Joseph, M., Verdieck, M., Zabora, J. and Fetting, J., (1993) "Spiritual Awareness, Personal Perspective on Death, and Psychosocial Distress Among Cancer Patients: An Initial Investigation", *Journal of Psychosocial Oncology,* 11,3:89-103.
Smith, R., (1982) "The Ethics of Ignorance", *Journal of Medical Ethics,*

18:117-118.
Smoot, G. and Davidson, K., (1993) *Wrinkles in Time,* Little Brown and Company, London.
Smyth, E., (ed.), (1991) *Postmodernism and Contemporary Fiction,* B T Batsford, London.
Soeken, K. and Carson, V., (1986) "Study Measures Nurses" Attitudes About Providing Spiritual Care", *Health Progress,* April:52-55.
Solzhenitsyn, A., (1971) *Cancer Ward,* Penguin Books, London.
Somerville, M., (1993) *The Song of Death: The Lyrics of Euthanasia,* The Catholic University of America.
Spiritual Care Work Group of the International Work Group on Death, Dying and Bereavement, (1990) "Assumptions and Principles of Spiritual Care", *Death Studies,* 14:75-81.
Stanley, D. and Reid, D., (1989) "Withholding Cardiopulmonary Resuscitation: One Hospital's Policy", *The Medical Journal of Australia,* 151,4/9:257-262.
Starr, P., (1979) "The Phantom Community", in *Co-ops, Communes and Collectives: Experiments in Social Change in the 1960s and 1970s,* Case, J. and Taylor, R., (eds.), Pantheon, New York.
Stepnick, A. and Perry, T., (1992) "Preventing Spiritual Distress in the Dying Patient", *Journal of Psychosocial Nursing,* 30,1:17-24.
Stiles, M., (1990) "The Shining Stranger: Nurse-family Spiritual Relationship", *Cancer Nursing,* 13,4:235-245.
Stoddard, S., (1979) *The Hospice Movement: A Better Way of Caring for the Dying,* Jonathan Cape, London.
Stuart, E., Deckro, J. and Mandle, C., (1989) "Spirituality in Health and Healing: A Clinical Program", *Holistic Nursing Practice,* 3,3:35-36.
Stuparich, J., (ed.), (1992) *Euthanasia, Palliative and Hospice Care and the Terminally Ill,* A Seminar held at John XXIII College Australian National University, Canberra.
Sudnow, D., (1967) *Passing On: The Social Organization of Dying,* Prentice-Hall, Englewood Cliffs, New Jersey.
Sutherland, C., (1992) *Transformed by the Light, Life After Near-Death Experience,* Bantam Books, Sydney.
Taussig, M., (1980) "Reification and the Consciousness of the Patient", *Social Science and Medicine,* 14b:3-13.
Taylor, E., (1993) "Factors Associated with Meaning in Life Among People with Recurrent Cancer", *Oncology Nursing Forum,* 20,9:1399-1407.
Taylor, E., Highfield, M. and Amenta, M., (1994) "Attitudes and Beliefs Regarding Spiritual Care", *Cancer Nursing,* 17,6:479-487.
Taylor, P. and Ferszt, G., (1990) "Spiritual Healing", *Holistic Nursing Practice,* 4,4:32-38.
Taylor, R., (1986) "The Four Phases of Prevention", *New Doctor,* 41/42:21-27.
Teo, B., (1991) "Organs for Transplantation, The Singapore Experience", *Hastings Center Report,* November/December:10-13.
Thomson, C., (1982) "Defining Death to Save Life: Legal and Ethical

Dilemmas of Tissue Transplants", *New Doctor,* 24:16-18.
Tomm, K., (1988) "Interventive Interviewing: Part 111. Intending to Ask Lineal, Circular, Strategic, or Reflexive Questions?", *Family Process,* 27,1:1-15.
Tomlinson, T. and Brody, H., (1988) "Ethics and Communication in Do-Not-Resuscitate Orders", *The New England Journal of Medicine,* 318,1:43-46.
Tonti-Filippini, N., (1992) "Some Refusals of Medical Treatment Which Changed the Law of Victoria", *The Medical Journal of Australia,* 157:277-279.
Torda, T. and Gerber, P., (1989) "To Resuscitate or Not, That is the Question", *The Medical Journal of Australia,* 1,4/9:243-245.
Townsend, J., Frank, A., Fermont, D., Dyer, S., Karran, O., Walgrove, A. and Piper, M., (1990) "Terminal Cancer and Patients" Preference for Place of Death: A Prospective Study", *British Medical Journal,* 301:415-417.
Truog, R., Brett, A. and Frader, J., (1992) "Sounding Board : The Problem With Futility", *The New England Journal of Medicine,* 326,23:1560-1563.
Turner, B., (1987) *Medical Power and Social Knowledge,* Sage Publications, London.
Turner, B., (1990) "The Interdisciplinary Curriculum: From Social Medicine to Postmodernsim", *Sociology of Health and Illness,* 12,1:2-23.
Vachon, M., (1983) "Staff Stress in Care of the Terminally Ill" in *Hospice Care: Principles and Practice,* Corr, C. and Corr, D., (eds.), Faber and Faber, New York.
Vachon, M., (1986) "Myths and Realities in Palliative/Hospice Care", in *Nursing in Hospice and Terminal Care: Research and Practice,* Petrosino, B., (ed.), The Haworth Press, London.
Vachon, M., (1993) "Emotional Problems in Palliative Medicine: Patient, Family, and Professional", in *Oxford Textbook of Palliative Medicine,* Doyl, D., Hanks, G. and Macdonald, N., (eds.), Oxford University Press, Oxford.
Valverde, M., (1991) "As If Subjects Existed: Analysing Social Discourses", *Canadian Review of Sociology and Anthropology,* 28,2:173-187.
Van Dijk, T. A., (1989) "Structures of Discourse and Structures of Power", in *Communication Yearbook 12,* Anderson, J., (ed.), Sage, Newbury Park, Ca.
Veatch, R., (1976) *Death, Dying and the Biological Revolution: Our Last Quest for Responsibility,* Yale University Press, New Haven.
Veatch, R., (1988) "Justice and the Economics of Terminal Illness" *Hastings Center Report,* 18/8:34-40.
Veatch, R., (ed.), (1989) *Medical Ethics,* Jones and Bartlett, Boston.
Waitzkin, H., (1989) "A Critical Theory of Medical Discourse: Ideology, Social Control and the Processing of Social context in Medical Encounters", *Journal of Health and Social Behaviour,* 30,(June):220-239.
Waitzkin, H. and Stoeckle, J., (1976) "Information Control and the Micropolitics of Health Care: Summary of an Ongoing Research Project",*Social Science and Medicine,* 10:263-276.
Wald, F., Foster, Z. and Wald, H., (1980) "The Hospice Movement as a Health Care Reform", *Nursing Outlook,* March:173-178.
Walker, Q., Gebski, V. and Lang, A., (1989) "The Misuse of Mammography in

the Management of Breast Cancer Revisited", *The Medical Journal of Australia,* 151,6/11:509-511.
Walsh, S., (1992) "A Patient's Story", *Clinical Trials - We Can"t Live Without Them,* Unpublished Paper, Ethics Seminar Friday 2nd October, Mater Misericordiae Public Hospitals, Brisbane.
Wanzer, S., Adelstein, J., Cranford, R., Federman, D., Hook, E., Moertel, C., Safar, P., Stone, A., Taussig, H. and Van Eys, J., (1984) "The Physician's Responsibility Toward Hopelessly Ill Patients", *The New England Journal of Medicine,* 310,15:955-959.
Ward, C., (1947) *Buddhism,* The Epworth Press, London.
Watts, A., (1971) *Eastern Wisdom - The Tao in China,* (audiocassette), The Center for Cassettes Studies.
Watts, I. and Price, S., (1995) "The Future of Palliative Care - Funding and Strategies", *Palliative Care Association of Queensland Seminar,* Mater Hospital, Brisbane.
Wear, A. and Brahams, D., (1991) "To Treat or Not To Treat: The Legal, Ethical and Therapeutic Implications of Treatment Refusal", *Journal of Medical Ethics,* 17:131-135.
Weber, M., (1958) *From Max Weber:Essays in Sociology,*Oxford University Press, New York.
Weedon, C., (1987) *Feminist Practice and Poststructuralist Theory,* Blackwell, Oxford.
Weigold, J., (1985) *Joy Against Cancer,* A Kevin Weldon Production, Australia.
Weiz, G., (1991) "Introduction" in *Social Science Perspectives on Medical Ethics*, Weisz, G., (ed.), University of Pennsylvania Press, Philadelphia.
Whyte, W., (1982) "Interviewing in Field Research", in *Field Research: A Sourcebook and Field Manual,* Burgess, R., (ed.), George Allen and Unwin, London.
Wiernik, P., (ed.), (1982) *Controversy in Oncology,* Wiley Medical Publication, New York.
Wildes, K., (1992) "Principles, Rules, Duties, and Babel: Bioethics in the Face of Postmodernity", *The Journal of Medicine and Philosophy,* 17:483-485.
Wilkinson, H., (1986) "Assessment of Patient Satisfaction and Hospice: A Review and an Investigation", *The Hospice Journal,*2,4:69-94.
Wilkinson, H., MacDonald, D. and Pilz, L., (1990) "Issues of Concern to Hospice Personnel: Results of a Hospice Opinion Poll", *The American Journal of Hospice and Palliative Care,* July/August:31-36.
Williams, A., (1974) "The Cost Benefit Approach", *British Medical Journal,* 30:252-256.
Williams, A., (1992) "Cost-Effectiveness Analysis: Is It Ethical?", *Journal of Medical Ethics,* 18:7-11.
Williams, B., (1972) *Morality: An Introduction to Ethics,* Cambridge University Press, Cambridge.
Williams, B., (1985) *Ethics and the Limits of Philosophy,* Fontana Press, London.
Williams, R., (1990) "Which Came First: The Hospice or the Funding?",

American Journal of Hospice and Palliative Care, 7,4:21-26.

Willis, E., (1989) *Medical Dominance,* Allen and Unwin, Sydney.

Willis, E., (1994) *Illness and Social Relations, Issues in the Sociology of Health Care,* Allen and Unwin, St Leonards, NSW.

Wilson, P., (1983) "Dying and Death of a Hospice in a Tertiary Hospital: Case History" in *Hospice USA,* Kutscher, A., Klagsbrun, S., Torpic, R., De Bellis, R., Hale, M. and Tallner, M., (eds.), Columbia University Press, New York.

Wilson, R., (1983) *The Sociology of Health: An Introduction,* Random House, New York.

Wolf, S. and Berle, B., (eds.), (1981) *The Technological Imperative in Medicine,* Plenum Press, New York.

Wolf, S., (1991) "Honoring Broader Directives", *Hastings Center Report, Special Supplement,* September-October:S8-S9.

Wong, E. and Lincoln, T., (1983) "Ready! Fire! Aim! An Inquiry into Laboratory Test Ordering", *Journal of the American Medical Association,* 250,11:2510-2513.

Worton, M. and Still, J., (eds.), (1990) *Intertextuality: Theories and Practices,* Manchester University Press, Manchester.

Wreen, M., (1991) "Autonomy, Religious Values, and Refusal of Lifesaving Medical Treatment", *Journal of Medical Ethics,* 17:124-130.

Zaner, R., (1990) "Medicine and Dialogue", *The Journal of Medicine and Philosophy,* 15:303-325.

Zerwekh, J., (1995) "A Family Caregiving Model for Hospice Nursing", *The Hospice Journal,* 10,(1):27-43.

Zimmerman, J., (1981) *Hospice: Complete Care for the Terminally Ill,* Urban and Schwarzenberg, Baltimore-Munich.

Zola, I., (1975) "In the Name of Health and Illness: On Some Socio-political Consequences of Medical Influence", *Social Science and Medicine,* 9:83-87.

Zola, I., (1979) "Pathways to the Doctor - From Person to Patient", in *Health, Illness, and Medicine,* Albrecht, G. and Higgins, P., Rand McNally, Chicago.

Zola, I., (1980) "Structural Constraints in the Doctor-Patient Relationship: The Case of Non-Compliance", *The Relevance of Social Science for Medicine,* Eisenberg, L. and Kleinman, A., (eds.), D Reidel Pub. Co., London.

Zola, I., (1990) "Medicine as an Institution of Social Control", in *Sociology of Health and Illness: Critical Perspectives,* Conrad, P. and Kern, R., (eds.), St Martin's Press, New York.

For Product Safety Concerns and Information please contact our EU representative GPSR@taylorandfrancis.com Taylor & Francis Verlag GmbH, Kaufingerstraße 24, 80331 München, Germany

Batch number: 10725923

Printed by Printforce, the Netherlands